"Ling and Hauck provide practical examples of the DO ART method for using art to engage in deliberative ethical decision making. Mental health practitioners have many resources at their disposal to ensure ethical practice. This book provides detailed examples to support art therapists endeavoring to utilize a creative art making process to resolve contemporary, cultural and contextual ethical dilemmas."

—**Cheryl Doby-Copeland, PhD, ATR-BC, LPC, LMFT,** *clinical program coordinator, Parent Infant Early Childhood Enhancement Program, honorary life member AATA*

"DO ART: is both an effective acronym and a great call to action. Dilemma; Outcome; Assistance; Responsibility and Take Action, with artmaking at each step, provides a pathway to practical and nuanced ethical decision making for art therapists. This unique collaborative book, lucidly written and soundly researched, demonstrates the DO ART process with vividly illustrated examples."

—**Dan Anthon, ATR-BC, LCPC,** *AATA Ethics Committee*

"The DO ART decision making tool, developed by the authors, is an innovative and thorough way to analyze ambiguous ethical dilemmas. This is particularly challenging in art therapy, where creative process, materials and visual symbolism add an integral layer to verbal treatment. A strength of this model is that art making plays a vital role in evaluating the ethical dilemmas and alternate outcomes. Case examples are thoroughly analyzed and range from cultural issues to doing artwork with sensitive populations. This text is especially relevant when it examines clinical situations unique to art therapy. Annotated bibliographies are featured at the end of each chapter, enabling readers to explore topics on a deeper level."

—**Laura V. Loumeau-May, MPS, ATR-BC, LPC**

"This book is a valuable addition to the art therapy literature and a helpful resource for art therapy educators and practitioners. The DO ART Model offers a practical, step-by-step template for thinking through difficult situations in clinical work and underscores potential ethical challenges that are unique to the practice of art therapy."

—**Marie Wilson, PhD, ATR-BC, ATCS,** *professor emerita, Caldwell University*

W0234772

Navigating Ethical Dilemmas in Creative Arts Therapies

Navigating Ethical Dilemmas in Creative Arts Therapies uses a case-based approach to provide practical guidance for practitioners on the skillful application of ethical decision-making in art therapy.

The book introduces the DO ART model, an ethical decision-making model specific to the practice of art therapy. Walking readers through common areas of ethical dilemmas, chapters detail how art-making can be used to navigate the model, supporting the well-documented practice of art therapists engaging in art-making processes themselves. Topics covered include boundaries and confidentiality, assessment, storage and exhibition, materials, multicultural issues, technology in art therapy, working with vulnerable populations, supervision and training, and ethical research.

Art therapists at all levels will find this book to be a necessary resource for their practice.

Thomson J. Ling, PhD, is a professor at Caldwell University where he has been teaching counseling and art therapy ethics for over a decade.

Jessica M. Hauck, MA, is an art therapist, mental health counselor, and adjunct professor, with expertise in ethical practice and numerous art therapy publications.

Navigating Ethical Dilemmas in Creative Arts Therapies

A Case-Based Approach

Edited by Thomson J. Ling and Jessica M. Hauck

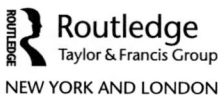
Routledge
Taylor & Francis Group

NEW YORK AND LONDON

First published 2022
by Routledge
605 Third Avenue, New York, NY 10158

and by Routledge
2 Park Square, Milton Park, Abingdon, Oxon, OX14 4RN

Routledge is an imprint of the Taylor & Francis Group, an informa business

© 2022 selection and editorial matter, Thomson J. Ling and Jessica M. Hauck; individual chapters, the contributors

Library of Congress Cataloging-in-Publication Data

Names: Ling, Thomson J., editor. | Hauck, Jessica M., editor.
Title: Navigating ethical dilemmas in creative arts therapies : a case-based approach / edited by Thomson J. Ling and Jessica M. Hauck.
Description: New York, NY : Routledge, 2022. | Includes bibliographical references and index. |
Identifiers: LCCN 2021034243 (print) | LCCN 2021034244 (ebook) | ISBN 9781032006727 (hardback) | ISBN 9781032006710 (paperback) | ISBN 9781003175124 (ebook)
Subjects: LCSH: Arts–Therapeutic use–Moral and ethical aspects.
Classification: LCC RC489.A72 N388 2022 (print) | LCC RC489.A72 (ebook) | DDC 616.89/1656–dc23/eng/20211029
LC record available at https://lccn.loc.gov/2021034243
LC ebook record available at https://lccn.loc.gov/2021034244

ISBN: 978-1-032-00672-7 (hbk)
ISBN: 978-1-032-00671-0 (pbk)
ISBN: 978-1-003-17512-4 (ebk)

DOI: 10.4324/9781003175124

Typeset in Times New Roman
by MPS Limited, Dehradun

Contents

Figures

Acknowledgments

Working on this book was a joy and incredible learning experience and would not have been possible without the tremendous support of many colleagues, mentors, friends, and family. I am grateful for the many students who have taken my legal and ethical issues in counseling class over the past decade. They have taught me a tremendous amount about teaching ethics and the professional development of therapists. Their questions, comments, and willingness to challenge my ideas inspired me to develop and refine the ethical decision-making model. I would like to acknowledge Sr. Catherine Waters who initially assigned me to teach a graduate course on ethics and encouraged me to seek excellence in ensuring the next generation of students had strong ethical decision-making skills.

Special thanks to Amanda Devine and Grace McDonnell at Routledge who saw the potential in this project and supported it along the way. I would also like to thank the chapter authors for their willingness to draw from their professional expertise and write about ethical dilemmas using the model.

My deepest thanks go to my co-editor and co-author, Jessica Hauck, for her collaboration, insight, dedication, and humor. It has been a pleasure collaborating with Jessica over the past six years and I look forward to many more projects. Finally, I thank my life partner, Allison Warner, for her unrelenting support. Her patience, contributions, and sacrifices make all things possible.

–**Thomson J. Ling**

I am extremely grateful for the support and guidance of so many people. First, I thank the contributors to this book, whose support and encouragement of ethical practice in the field of art therapy cannot be understated, and whose chapters made it possible to share this model.

I also give very special thanks to Taylor & Francis for supporting this project in its earliest drafts, and express my sincere gratitude to Amanda Devine and Grace McDonnell, for their encouragement and editorial support. My professional development has been supported by so many wonderful colleagues, teachers, and supervisors, along with the training I received at Caldwell University. I am especially grateful for the support and encouragement of my mentor, Thomson Ling, without whom this book would not have been possible.

My grandparents have always been supportive of my academic and writing pursuits, and I'm so grateful to my Pop-Pop Raoul for his advice and encouragement. I also need to thank my incredible husband, Mike, for his endless patience and amazing sense of humor. Finally, thanks to my parents and sister, for their love and support.

–**Jessica M. Hauck**

List of Abbreviations

AATA   American Art Therapy Association
ATCB   Art Therapy Credentials Board

Contributors

Amanda Bezold, Caldwell University, Caldwell, NJ

Jongwon Melissa Choi, Caldwell University, Caldwell, NJ

Miki Goerdt, LCSW, ATR-BC, Emerald Leaf Counseling LLC, VA

Jessica M. Hauck, MA, LAC, ATR-P, Caldwell University, Caldwell, NJ

Erin Hein, ATR-BC, LPC, St. Luke's Medical Center & Aurora Sinai Hospital, Milwaukee, WI

Laura Holland, MA, LAC, ATR-P, Caldwell University, Caldwell, NJ

Thomson J. Ling, PhD, Caldwell University, Caldwell, NJ

Michele Marotta, Caldwell University, Caldwell, NJ

Jill McNutt, PhD, ATR-BC, ATRL, LPC, ATCS, Saint Mary-of-the-Woods College, Saint Mary of the Woods, IN

Jenna Park, MA, Caldwell University, Caldwell, NJ

Jenna Pattison, Caldwell University, Caldwell, NJ

Melanie A. Peters, MA, ATR-BC, LAC, Atlantic Health System, NJ

Mary Ellen Ruff, PhD, LPC, ATR-BC, ACS, George Washington University, Washington, DC

Victoria Scarborough, MPS, ATR-BC, LPC-AT-S, CEDS

Patricia A. St John Tager, EdD, ATR-BC, LCAT, College of New Rochelle, New Rochelle, NY

Faith Thayer, PhD, LPC, LCAT, ATR-BC

Monica Wright, MA, LAC, Caldwell University, Caldwell, NJ

1 Introduction to Ethical Issues in Creative Art Therapies

Jessica M. Hauck and Thomson J. Ling

Art therapy is a unique branch of the helping professions. The American Art Therapy Association (2017) defines art therapy as "an integrative mental health and human services profession that enriches the lives of individuals, families, and communities through active art-making, creative process, applied psychological theory, and human experience within a psychotherapeutic relationship." This places art therapy as a unique intersection between verbal, visual, and kinesthetic therapeutic interventions. While art therapy provides a unique and comprehensive treatment approach, it also creates challenges in ethical practice. As with all therapeutic interventions, ethical practice in art therapy is of profound importance and literature has elucidated the harm unethical art therapy can cause clients (e.g., Furman, 2013; Moon & Nolan, 2020; Sprigham, 2008).

In recent years, the importance of ethical art therapy practice has been demonstrated through an increase in research and literature (e.g., Hinz, 2013, 2017; Kaiser, 2016, 2017; Kapitan, 2011; Karcher, 2017; Molloy, 2017; Talwar, 2017; Zappa, 2017). Twice, Art Therapy: Journal of the American Art Therapy Association has dedicated an issue to the topic of ethics: in 2011 an issue was focused on ethical challenges (Kapitan, 2011), and in 2017 an issue was dedicated to ethics and cultural competence (Talwar, 2017). In addition, the American Art Therapy Association's Annual Conference has included ethics as a topic of perennial interest (e.g., Agell & Goodman, 1995; McAlevey et al., 2016; Robb et al., 2015). Multiple books have been written on ethical issues in art therapy (e.g., Moon & Nolan, 2020; Furman, 2013; Farrant et al., 2014; DiMaria, 2019). Further, the art therapy literature has also extensively discussed ethics, covering topics such as positive approaches to ethics (Hinz, 2011, 2017), ethics and cultural competence (Kaiser, 2016), foster care (Molloy, 2017), ethical treatment of art therapy images (Hinz, 2013), social justice (e.g., Kaiser, 2017; Karcher, 2017; Zappa, 2017), social media in art therapy (Alders et al., 2015; Belkofer & McNutt, 2011), the exhibition of artwork (Vick, 2011), art therapy with specific populations and settings (e.g., Furman, 2011; Moriya, 2011), the conduct of research in art therapy (Deaver, 2011), and the practice of pro bono art therapy (Moon, 2011).

DOI: 10.4324/9781003175124-1

1.1 Common Issues in the Ethical Practice of Art Therapy

Some ethical issues that art therapists face overlap with other helping professions. For example, the practice of art therapy involves working with diverse populations. Indeed, art therapists' ethical principles include multicultural and diversity competence (American Art Therapy Association, 2013) and the American Art Therapy Association has promoted multicultural competence through formal initiatives (Potash et al., 2015). Yet, literature has indicated that increased diversity is needed in this field (Awais & Yali, 2015). While multicultural competence is an important part of all clinical work, the specific ethical issues surrounding multicultural competence are unique for art therapists. For example, art therapists must be cognizant of ensuring access to culturally diverse materials (e.g., paints and other art materials often do not represent all skin tones). In addition to materials, art therapists also need to take care to ensure that the techniques they use honor the cultural origins from which they are borrowed (e.g., using mandalas in therapy).

Ethical practice with populations is especially important when it comes to working with vulnerable populations. Typically, vulnerable populations refer to children, prisoners, pregnant women, mentally disabled persons, or economically or educationally disadvantaged persons. While the literature is somewhat limited in this area, art therapists should be sure to follow all relevant laws and regulations. One issue that has been identified in the literature, which relates to working with vulnerable populations, is the use of the third-hand technique, first developed by Edith Kramer (Kramer, 1986). This technique can be thought of as a way of intervening therapeutically and should be used to support or enhance a client's creative development, without being intrusive. It may be done verbally (e.g., cautioning a client that their hand may smudge the paper if they continue) or physically (e.g., holding a client's clay figure together while they reinforce it). The issue of when to intervene or when not to intervene is directly related to several aspirational principles for art therapists, including client autonomy. However, the issues surrounding the ethical practice of art therapy with vulnerable populations transcend issues of client autonomy.

Aside from issues that overlap with other helping professions, there are also ethical issues specific to art therapy. As a growing profession, the ethical supervision and training of new professionals are of utmost importance in the field. Art therapist supervisors are responsible for ensuring that all those who supervise and train are practicing ethically and within their bounds of competence. Important general ethical issues to consider include navigating dual relationships and disclosing personal information. More specific to art therapy, the use of response art in supervision (Fish 2006, 2012), a commonly used technique, should also be approached carefully (Deaver & Shiflett, 2011). Likewise, while all helping professions include maintaining healthy boundaries and ensuring confidentiality as central tenets of ethical practice, these issues are often magnified in the field of art therapy. For example, the American Art Therapy Association's (2013) Ethical Principles discuss the ethical exhibition of client artwork and requires art therapists to take extra steps to maintain confidentiality. Similarly, art therapists are often involved with the art community and this creates possibilities for multiple relationships.

Another aspect of art therapy educational training is the ethical research practices, which include both conducting research (Anderson, 2001) but also interpreting and applying research to practice (Kaiser et al., 2006). However, what constitutes good research has been discussed by the literature (Deaver, 2002). For example, art therapy research tends to focus on qualitative methodologies and case studies. Consequently, research has suggested that the need for studies that demonstrate art therapy effectiveness is needed (Slayton et al., 2010). Without a strong research foundation, art therapists may unethically engage in practices that have little to no support. Further, without proper training, art therapists may misinterpret research findings.

In today's world, technology and technology-assisted services are being utilized more and more to provide therapeutic services for individuals who are unable or unwilling to attend in-person treatment. These telehealth services can be incredibly beneficial for clients, and increase access to those who may otherwise have gone without, but they also come with a variety of ethical concerns. This includes determining/verifying the identity of the client, maintaining confidentiality, and following licensure and legal requirements for the state(s) where both the client and art therapist reside (American Art Therapy Association, 2013). Clients should also be provided with informed consent regarding how the session is being documented and if it's being recorded. Telehealth can be difficult to navigate for all helping professions, but with art therapy, ethical issues may be magnified. These include, but are not limited to, access to art materials and a safe and confidential workspace.

More recently, art therapists have begun to embrace digital mediums in the practice of art therapy. The use of digital art in the therapeutic process has both benefits and drawbacks, which should be carefully addressed with clients before incorporating its use in treatment. For some clients, especially those with sensory issues, it can open up a world of opportunity for treatment. But for others, it may be inundating them with an unnecessary amount of screen time and distancing them from the overall process and hands-on therapeutic benefit. These concerns raise important questions on how and when to use various art-making methods in art therapy treatment.

Art therapists are well aware of the importance of access to art materials in art therapy. Art materials range on a continuum from fluid to rigid, with different types of materials eliciting different reactions from clients. Fluid art materials provide less control, but more flexibility.

However, they may be over-stimulating, and cause clients to regress. Rigid art materials provide more control, but less flexibility. Clients may view rigid art materials as safer than fluid art materials, but they may also be too restricting or under-stimulating. Careful consideration should be used to determine which types of materials are most appropriate for which client, in which situations (American Art Therapy Association, 2013). It is important to consider sensory sensitivities, fine motor skills, and culturally appropriate/inclusive materials. Other ethical concerns may relate to the use of the materials themselves, including how to effectively work with clients that are resistant toward certain materials, or insist on taking more than is needed of others (e.g., using too much paint, breaking charcoals). The gathering of materials also brings its own ethical challenges, as many agencies are unable to maintain a significant budget for art materials, and instead rely on donations.

Art therapy treatment methods may include a focus on process, the finished product, or both. Art-based assessment, which traditionally focuses more on a product, has continued to gain popularity over the years, with new tools being developed and existing tools being assessed for reliability and validity. As with any assessment, there are ethical concerns that should be addressed, especially as it relates to the selection, administration, and interpretation of various art-based assessment tools (American Art Therapy Association, 2013). For example, a principle of art therapy assessments is that artwork should never be formally used to assess a client if it wasn't created in front of the art therapist.

Many art therapists stand behind the idea that art is a record and should be treated as such. Certain ethical concerns surrounding this issue are likely to come up during practice, whether the art therapist is working in private practice, at a small community agency, or at a larger hospital setting, etc. Unlike most medical records, which are typically easy to store and maintain, the art created during art therapy sessions can be much more difficult to preserve. Care must be taken to ensure the artwork is undamaged and protected from possible breaches of confidentiality. This process may include photographing art that is too difficult to keep, or maintaining a storage system where the art can be kept in a temperature-controlled and private setting. Art therapy treatment records for clients should typically be kept for the amount of time dictated by federal, state, and institutional laws then are disposed of in a way that maintains confidentiality (American Art Therapy Association, 2013). Ethical guidelines also explain that artwork may be released to the client during the course of treatment or during the termination process, and that clients should provide informed consent if records of the art are being kept. Artwork created during the session belongs to the client(s) that created it. Exhibiting this artwork can be a great opportunity to decrease stigma, build confidence and empower the client, and build awareness of the profession as a whole (Vick, 2011) however also carries unique challenges.

These may include possible breaches of confidentiality as well as other impacts to the client's emotional well-being, especially if the artwork being exhibited is also for sale.

1.2 Ethical Codes and Principles

Consistent with all health professions, art therapists practice within an ethical framework. The *Ethical Principles for Art Therapists* (American Art Therapy Association, 2013) and the recently updated *Art Therapy Credentials Board Code of Professional Practice* (Art Therapy Credentials Board, 2021) are both guiding rules for the ethical practice of art therapy. These codes and principles provide a clear solution when situations are straightforward; however, in more complicated situations the most ethical solution is less clear (e.g., Furman, 2013; Kapitan, 2011). Indeed, the *Ethical Principles for Art Therapists* explicitly state, in principle 17.0, that the ethical "principles are written to provide a basis for education and a foundation for ethical practice" (American Art Therapy Association, 2013, p. 14). As such, these ethical guidelines are not entirely prescriptive, and different aspects of the ethical codes and principles may contradict each other, each suggesting different courses of action.

Complicating matters further, art therapists have long debated over their professional identities, with many identifying as artists in addition to art therapists. The necessity of multiple professional identities is evident by the fact that a majority of states do not provide a clear path for licensure as an art therapist. Only a handful of states provide art therapy specific licenses (e.g., Kentucky, Maryland, Mississippi, New Jersey, and New Mexico) and five additional states allow for art therapists to gain licensure under related areas (New York, Pennsylvania, Texas, Utah, and Washington) (Rastogi, 2017). Research has underscored this by illuminating common challenges art therapists face in training, including how art therapy and other creative modalities intersect with mental health counseling (e.g., Degges-White & Davis, 2011; McNiff, 2009; Van Lith & Voronin, 2016). Likewise, the question of how using creativity in counseling intersects with art therapy has been examined (Rosen & Atkins, 2014). Suffice to say that ethical decision-making in art therapy may involve blending multiple codes, principles, and professions.

1.3 Theories of Ethics that Should be Considered

One area of common ground may be in identifying the various theoretical bases that can be applied to ethical decision-making. Ideally, ethical decision-making considers a multitude of perspectives to arrive at the most ethical course of action (Corey et al., 2015; Remley & Herlihy, 2016; Welfel, 2016). While many models incorporate some of these ethical perspectives, we have found that few combine multiple perspectives into one decision-making model. There are three theories commonly used in ethical decision-making: utilitarianism, moral relativism, and deontological.

First, utilitarianism (sometimes referred to as teleological contextualism) suggests therapists consider how actions would lead to the greatest good for the greatest number of clients (Mills, 1863/2004; Warburton, 2013, p. 115). Using a utilitarianism perspective, therapists prioritize the consequences of a course of action rather than the manner in which the consequences are achieved.

Second, moral relativism places ethical decisions within a societal context (Sumner, 1906/2008; Warburton, 2013, p. 147). Moral relativism is sometimes used synonymously with antinomianism where art therapists are asked to consider the uniqueness of each situation. We apply this theory by suggesting that ethical actions should be based on industry-standard practices (i.e., what most therapists would do). For instance, current best practices consider the multicultural context of a situation (Frame & Williams, 2005). Moral relativism encourages therapists to seek assistance from others in the field to determine what are the industry standards that apply to a situation. Moral relativism also suggests that therapists educate themselves using literature relevant to the ethical situation in question.

Finally, unlike antinomianism, deontological legalism considers absolutist morals (Alexander & Moore, 2015; Kant, 1785/2004). This approach suggests that art therapists consider the rules and regulations over consequences in a situation. A deontological framework suggests consideration of liability and what actions in an ethical dilemma would serve to increase or limit therapists' exposure to liability.

1.4 Components of Ethical Decision-making Models

While all models lead to improved decision-making, there are many components that need to be considered in the selection of a decision-making model. First, models should be accessible and appropriate for practitioners of all experience levels (e.g., Hauck & Ling, 2016; Sileo & Kopala, 1993). Due to the nebulous nature of some ethical decision-making models, some are only appropriate for more experienced practitioners. Some models, such as those developed by Forester-Miller and Davis (1996; Stone, 2009), ask practitioners to consider specific codes of ethics but do not explain the details or include case examples for demonstration. Other models require therapists to consider specific issues for which they lack prerequisite knowledge, such as faculty-student dual relationships (Hill & Mamalakis, 2001). This may be problematic given the limited ethical training practitioners receive (Neukrug & Milliken, 2011).

Next, since industry standards change over time, models should provide flexibility and adaptability to new or updated ethical codes. For example, some existing models, like the one created by Stone (2009), are only appropriate for one specific code of ethics. Good ethical decision-making should allow for the use and application of multiple codes of ethics (e.g., American Counseling Association, 2014a, 2014b; American Art Therapy Association, 2013). In addition, models should provide flexibility and adaptability to new or updated ethical codes. It is also important for ethical decision-making to consider recent relevant research and literature as it applies to a situation.

Third, addressing multicultural issues is particularly important in ethical decision-making because the AATA Ethical Principles require that practitioners do not engage in discrimination and ensure their practice is guided by the American Art Therapy Association's Art Therapy Multicultural and Diversity Competencies (American Art Therapy Association, 2013). Consequently, this requires that therapists consider the role of diversity as they make ethical decisions (American Art Therapy Association, 2011; Frame & Williams, 2005). Indeed, recent court cases have underscored the importance of multicultural competence (e.g., Behnke, 2012; Keeton v. Anderson-Wiley, 2011; Ward v. Wilbanks, 2010). Thus, having a model that is applicable to multicultural considerations is paramount.

Finally, some ethical decision-making models are only appropriate for a narrow scope of situations. Given that therapists may encounter a variety of situations, we believe that a broadly applicable model that can be used with a wide scope of cases simplifies how counselors approach situations (e.g., Hauck & Ling, 2016; Sileo & Kopala, 1993). Thus, eliminating the need to determine what model is most appropriate for any given case. Some ethical decision-making models are only appropriate for a narrow range of situations. For example, models by Biaggio et al. (1997), and Hill & Mamalakis (2001) only focused on dual relationships.

While many ethical decision-making models incorporate some of the abovementioned components until recently none incorporated all these components. As a result, the application of existing models of ethical decision-making to real-world scenarios may yield inconsistent actions by practitioners. Given that practitioners may encounter a variety of situations, we believe that a broadly applicable model that can be used with a wide range of cases simplifies how counselors approach situations. This eliminates the need to determine what model is most appropriate for any given case.

1.5 Existing Models

To aid in ethical practice, health professions have developed a variety of decision-making models (e.g., Corey et al., 2015; Forester-Miller & Davis, 1996; Frame & Williams, 2005; Hill & Mamalakis, 2001; Sileo & Kopala, 1993). These models tend to have common elements, but may cater to different specific populations or issues. Further, many of these models are dated and were created before the current AATA Principles. In addition, some models are designed for use with a narrow scope of cases (e.g., American School Counselor Association, 2009; Stone, 2009). Research has shown that current models may not yield comprehensive answers, may not lead to improved ethical decision-making, and are not theoretically grounded (Cottone & Claus, 2000; Barnett et al., 2007). This is especially troubling given research has shown that less than half of therapists report participating in an ethics-specific course as part of their ethics education (Neukrug & Milliken, 2011). Indeed, researchers have noted that there is a need for ethics training, particularly as related to ethical decision-making (Hill, 2004; Levitt et al., 2015). As a result, many ethical decision-making models do not result in consistent decision-making when applied by different practitioners to a situation (Haas et al., 1986; Woody, 2013). Having a model that is theoretically grounded, approachable, consider relevant literature, is widely applicable, and leads to consistent decision-making would be beneficial to counselors at all levels of experience.

1.6 Adding Art to Ethical Decision-Making

Ethical decision-making is often challenging for clinicians. However, research has shown that art-making is beneficial for art therapists as well as art therapy clients (e.g., Bucciarelli, 2016; Deaver & Shiflett, 2011; Fish, 2012; Markin et al., 2013; Moon, 2011). Further, it may be helpful as a mechanism to engage in the decision-making process effectively (Naumburg, 1966; Marshall, 2007). Consequently, it is beneficial to include directives in an ethical decision-making process as this allows art therapists to use their strengths in visual and verbal processing (Moon, 2011; Simon & Graham, 2005).

1.7 Ethical Decision-Making Models for Art Therapy

While it is clear that understanding ethical decision making in art therapy is an absolute necessity, it was only recently that a model developed for art therapists emerged (DO ART Model; Hauck & Ling, 2016, 2020). This model was developed with art making in mind and allows art therapists to take a positive stance in ethical decision-making (Hinz, 2011). The DO ART model was designed to reduce ambiguity and lead to overall improved ethical decision-making and represents one of the first ethical decision-making models in the helping professions to be evaluated for its effectiveness (Ling et al., 2019).

Drawing from the multitude of theoretical perspectives, the DO ART model combines utilitarianism, moral relativism and deontological legalism. Specifically, utilitarianism is used as the driving perspective in considering the various outcomes (both positive and negative) that might result as art therapists work to resolve ethical situations. Moral relativism is applied by seeking assistance from others in the field as well as using literature to determine the industry standards that apply to a situation. Finally, deontological legalism is used to consider what actions in an ethical dilemma would serve to increase or limit the liability exposure.

1.8 About this Book

This book will assist practitioners in mastering ethical decision-making. While some readers may be familiar with ethical decision-making, less than half of clinicians' report is completing an ethics-specific course as part of their formal education (Neukrug & Milliken, 2011). Further, research has found that the complexity of ethical decision-making calls for additional training (Hill, 2004; Levitt et al., 2015). This proposed book will provide practical guidance for practitioners on the skillful application of ethical decision-making in art therapy using a case-based approach.

The next chapter will introduce readers to the DO ART model and includes an explanation of how ethical decision-making can combine both verbal and visual modalities. The subsequent chapters will walk readers through common issues in the ethical practice of art therapy. Specifically, this book will cover navigating multiple professional identities, the ethics of art materials, boundaries and confidentiality, assessment, record-keeping, multicultural issues, technology in art therapy, working with vulnerable populations, supervision and training, and research. Each chapter will start with an overview of the ethical topic and its importance. Next, a de-identified case vignette and an analysis of the case using the DO ART ethical decision-making model will be provided. To aid readers in combining verbal and visual modalities, examples of art will also be included. A summary of the main concerns related to the ethical topic and tips for avoiding pitfalls will follow. Finally, a brief annotated bibliography of suggested further readings on the topic will conclude each chapter. The book will end with a discussion of the importance of practitioners adopting the principles and strategies of ethical decision-making throughout their practice as well as strategies for the mastery of ethical decision-making in creative art therapies.

References

Agell, G., & Goodman, R. (1995). The professional relationships: Ethics. *American Journal of Art Therapy*, *33*(4), 99–110. http://search.ebscohost.com/login.aspx?direct=true&db=fth&AN=9505240022&site=ehost-live

Alders, A., Beck, L., Allen, P. B., & Mosinski, B. (2015). Technology in art therapy: Ethical challenges. *Art Therapy: Journal of the American Art Therapy Association*, *28*(4), 165–170. 10.1080/07421656.2011.622683

Alexander, L., & Moore, M. (2015). Deontological ethics. In E. N. Zalta (Ed.), *The Stanford encyclopedia of philosophy*. Stanford University. http:// plato.stanford.edu/archives/spr2015/entries/ethics-deontological

American Counseling Association. (2014a). *2014 ACA code of ethics*. https:// www.counseling.org/docs/default-source/default-document-library/2014-code-of-ethics-finaladdress.pdf?sfvrsn=96b532c_2

American Counseling Association. (Producer). (2014b). *HT047: The new 2014 code of ethics: An overview* [Audio podcast]. http://www.counseling.org/ knowledge-center/podcasts/docs/default-source/aca-podcasts/ht043---the-new-2 014-code-of-ethics-an-overview

American Art Therapy Association. (2011). *Art therapy multicultural/diversity competencies*. https://arttherapy.org/wp-content/uploads/2017/06/Multicultural-Competencies.pdf

American Art Therapy Association. (2013). *Ethical principles for art therapists*. https://arttherapy.org/wp-content/uploads/2017/06/Ethical-Principles-for-Art-Therapists.pdf

American Art Therapy Association. (2017). *Definition of the profession*. https:// www.arttherapy.org/upload/2017_DefinitionofProfession.pdf

American School Counselor Association (2009). *School counseling principles: Ethics and law* (2nd ed.) https://www.schoolcounselor.org/getmedia/f041cbd0-7004-47a5-ba01-3a5d657c6743/Ethical-Standards.pdf

Anderson, F. E. (2001). Benefits of conducting research. *Art Therapy: Journal of the American Art Therapy Association, 18*(3), 134–141. 10.1080/07421656.2001 .10129733

Art Therapy Credentials Board. (2021). *Code of ethics, conduct, and disciplinary procedures*. https://www.atcb.org/wp-content/uploads/2020/07/ATCB-Code-of-Ethics-Conduct-DisciplinaryProcedures.pdf

Awais, Y. J. & Yali, A. M. (2015). Efforts in increasing racial and ethnic diversity in the field of art therapy. *Art Therapy: Journal of the American Art Therapy Association, 32*(3), 112–119. 10.1080/07421656.2015.1060842

Barnett, J. E., Behnke, S. H., Rosenthal, S. L., & Koocher, G. P. (2007). In case of ethical dilemma, break glass: Commentary on ethical decision making in practice. *Professional Psychology: Research and Practice, 38*(1), 7–12. 10.1037/ 0735-7028.38.1.7

Behnke, S. H. (2012). Constitutional claims in the context of mental health training: Religion, sexual orientation, and tensions between the first amendment and professional ethics, *Training and Education in Professional Psychology, 6*, 189–195. 10.1037/a0030809

Belkofer, C. M., & McNutt, J. M. (2011). Understanding social media culture and its ethical challenges for art therapist. *Art Therapy: Journal of the American Art Therapy Association, 28*(4), 159–164. 10.1080/07421656.2011.622684

Biaggio, M., Paget, T. L., & Chenoweth, M. S. (1997). A model for ethical management of faculty—Student dual relationships. *Professional psychology: Research and practice, 28*(2), 184. 10.1037/0735-7028.28.2.184

Bucciarelli, A. (2016). Art therapy: A transdisciplinary approach. *Art Therapy: Journal of the American Art Therapy Association, 33*(3), 151–155. 10.1080/ 07421656.2016.1199246

Corey, G., Corey, M. S., & Callanan, P. (2015). *Issues and ethics in the helping professions* (9th ed.). Brooks/Cole.

Cottone, R. R., & Claus, R. E. (2000). Ethical decision-making models: A review of the literature. *Journal of Counseling and Development, 78*(3), 275–283. 10.1002/j.1556-6676.2000.tb01908.x

Deaver, S. (2002). What constitutes art therapy research? *Art Therapy: Journal of the American Art Therapy Association, 19*(1), 23–27. 10.1080/07421656.2002.10129721

Deaver, S. P. (2011). Research ethics: Institutional review board oversight of art therapy research. *Art Therapy: Journal of the American Art Therapy Association, 28*(4), 171–176. 10.1080/07421656.2011.622685

Deaver, S., & Shiflett, C. (2011). Art-based supervision techniques. *The Clinical Supervisor 30*(2), 257–276. 10.1080/07325223.2011.619456

Degges-White, S., & Davis, N. L. (2011). *Integrating the expressive arts into counseling practice: Theory-based interventions.* Springer.

DiMaria, A. (2019). *Exploring ethical dilemmas in art therapy: 50 clinicians from 20 countries share their stories.* Routledge

Farrant, C., Pavlicevic, M., & Tsiris, G. (2014). *A guide to research ethics for art therapists and arts & health practitioners.* Jessica Kingsley Publishers.

Fish, B. J. (2006). *Image-based narrative inquiry of response art in art therapy* (UMI No. 3228081) [Doctoral dissertation, Union Institute and University]. Proquest Dissertations Publishing. https://www.proquest.com/openview/e02f323b27c47f6ce9420633d6e5b3b5/1?pq-origsite=gscholar&cbl=18750&diss=y

Fish, B. J. (2012). Response art: The art of the art therapist. *Art Therapy: Journal of the American Art Therapy Association, 29*(3), 138–143. 10.1080/07421656.2012.701594

Forester-Miller, H., & Davis, T. (1996). *A practitioner's guide to ethical decision making.* American Counseling Association. http://www.counseling.org/docs/ethics/practitioners_guide.pdf?sfvrsn=2

Frame, M. W., & Williams, C. B. (2005). A model of ethical decision making from a multicultural perspective. *Counseling and Values, 49*(3), 165–179. 10.1002/j.2161-007X.2005.tb01020.x

Furman, L. R. (2011). Last breath: Art therapy with a lung cancer patient facing imminent death. *Art Therapy: Journal of the American Art Therapy Association, 28*(4), 177–180. 10.1080/07421656.2011.622690

Furman, L. R. (2013). *Ethics in art therapy: Challenging topics for a complex modality.* Jessica Kingsley Publisher.

Hauck, J., & Ling, T. (2016). The DO ART model: An ethical decision-making model applicable to art therapy. *Art Therapy: Journal of the American Art Therapy Association, 33*(4), 203–208. 10.1080/07421656.2016.1231544

Hauck, J. M. & Ling, T. J. (2020). Applying art therapy directives to ethical decision-making. *Art Therapy: Journal of the American Art Therapy Association. 37*(1), 34–41. 10.1080/07421656.2019.1667669

Haas, L. J., Malouf, J. L., & Mayerson, N. H. (1986). Ethical dilemmas in psychological practice: Results of a national survey. *Professional psychology: Research and practice, 17*(4), 316–321. 10.1037/0735-7028.17.4.316

Hill, A. L. (2004). Ethics education: Recommendations for an evolving discipline. *Counseling and Values, 48*, 183–203. 10.1002/j.2161-007X.2004.tb00245.x

Hill, M. R., & Mamalakis, P. M. (2001). Family therapists and religious communities: Negotiating dual relationships. *Family Relations, 50*(3), 199–208. 10.1111/j.1741-3729.2001.00199.x

Hinz, L. D. (2011). Embracing excellence: A positive approach to ethical decision making. *Art Therapy: Journal of the American Art Therapy Association, 28*(4), 185–188. 10.1080/07421656.2011.622693

Hinz, L. D. (2013). The life cycle of images: Revisiting the ethical treatment of the art therapy image. *Art Therapy: Journal of the American Art Therapy Association, 30*(1), 46–49. 10.1080/07421656.2013.757757

Hinz, L. D. (2017). The ethics of art therapy: Promoting creativity as a force for positive change. *Art Therapy: Journal of the American Art Therapy Association, 34*(3), 142–145. 10.1080/07421656.2017.1343073

Kaiser, D. (2016). Ethics, law, and cultural competence in art therapy. *Art Therapy: Journal of the American Art Therapy Association, 33*(4), 217. 10.1080/07421656.2016.1268457

Kaiser, D. (2017). What do structural racism and oppression have to do with scholarship, research, and practice in art therapy? *Art Therapy: Journal of the American Art Therapy Association, 34*(3), 154–156. 10.1080/07421656.2017.1420124

Kaiser, D., St. John, P., & Ball, B. (2006). Teaching art therapy research: A brief report. *Art Therapy: Journal of the American Art Therapy Association, 23*(4), 186–190.

Kapitan, L. (2011). "But is it ethical?" Articulating an art therapy ethos. *Art Therapy: Journal of the American Art Therapy Association, 28*(4), 150–151. 10.1080/07421656.2011.624930

Kant, I. (2004). *Fundamental principles of the metaphysic of morals.* T. K. Abbott (Trans.). http://www.gutenberg.org/cache/epub/5682/pg5682-images.html (Original work published 1785)

Karcher, O. P. (2017). Sociopolitical oppression, trauma, and healing: Moving toward a social justice art therapy framework. *Art Therapy: Journal of the American Art Therapy Association, 34*(3), 123–128. 10.1080/07421656.2017.1358024

Keeton v. Anderson-Wiley. (2011). 664 F. 3d 865.

Kramer, E. (1986). The art therapist's third hand: Reflections on art, art therapy, and society at large. *American Journal of Art Therapy. 24*(3), 71–86.

Levitt, D. H., Farry, T. J., & Mazzarella, J. R. (2015). Counselor ethical reasoning: Decision-making practice versus theory. *Counseling and Values, 60,* 84–99. 10.1002/j.2161-007X.2015.00062.x

Ling, T. J., Hauck, J. M., Doyle, C. J., Percario, K. N., & Henawi, T. (2019). Evaluating the use of ethical decision-making models for art therapy. *Art Therapy: Journal of the American Art Therapy Association. 36*(2), 93–97. 10.1080/07421656.2019.1609330

McAlevey, M. E., Anand, S. A., & Towne, T. (2016). *ATCB code of ethics, professional practice, and disciplinary procedures: What's new.* Panel discussion at the American Art Therapy Association Annual Conference, Baltimore, MD.

McNiff, S. (2009). *Integrating the arts in therapy: History, theory and practice.* Charles C. Thomas.

Markin, R. D., McCarthy, K. S., & Barber, J. P. (2013). Transference, counter-transference, emotional expression, and session quality over the course of supportive expressive therapy: The rater's perspective. *Psychotherapy Research, 23*, 152–168. 10.1080/10503307/2012.747013

Marshall, J. (2007). Image as insight: Visual images in practice-based research. *Studies in Art Education, 49*(1), 23–41. 10.1080/00393541.2007.11518722

Mills, J. S. (2004). *Utilitarianism.* http://www.gutenberg.org/files/11224/11224-h/11224-h.htm (Original work published 1863)

Molloy, J. N. (2017). Post-ASFA permanency planning for children in foster care: Clinical and ethical considerations for art therapists. *Art Therapy: Journal of the American Art Therapy Association, 34*(3), 102–105. 10.1080/07421656.2017.1353334

Moon, B. L. (2011). Ethical dilemmas of providing pro bono art therapy. *Art Therapy: Journal of the American Art Therapy Association, 28*(4), 180–184. 10.1080/07421656.2011.622696

Moon, B. L., & Nolan, E. G. (2020). *Ethical issues in art therapy* (4th ed.). Charles C. Thomas.

Moriya, D. (2011). Ethical issues in school art therapy. *Art Therapy: Journal of the American Art Therapy Association, 28*(4), 59–65. 10.1080/07421656.2006.10129643

Naumburg, M. (1966). *Dynamically oriented art therapy: Its principles and practices, illustrated with three case studies.* Grune & Stratton.

Neukrug, E., & Milliken, T. (2011). Counselors' perceptions of ethical behaviors. *Journal of Counseling and Development, 89*, 206–216. 10.1002/j.1556-6678.2011.tb00079.x

Potash, J. S., Doby-Copeland, C., Stepney, S. A., Washington, B. N., Vance, L. D., Short, G. M., Boston, C. G., & ter Maat, M. (2015). Advancing multicultural and diversity competence in art therapy: American Art Therapy Association Multicultural Committee 1990-2015. *Art Therapy: Journal of the American Art Therapy Association, 32*(3), 146–150. 10.1080/07421656.2015.1060837

Rastogi, M. (2017). *Creating a successful career in art therapy: Advising guide for psychology faculty and students.* https://teachpsych.org/resources/Documents/otrp/resources/Advising%20Guide%20for%20Art%20Therapy-edited4.docx

Remley, T. P., & Herlihy, B. (2016). *Ethical, legal, and professional issues in counseling* (5th ed.). Pearson.

Robb, M., Deaver, S., Potash, J., & Furman, L. (2015, July). *What are current ethical practices in research?* Panel discussion presented at the American Art Therapy Association Annual Conference, Minneapolis, MN. http://www.arttherapy.org/upload/2015onlineconferencebrochure.pdf

Rosen, C. M., & Atkins, S. S. (2014). Am I doing expressive arts therapy or creativity in counseling? *Journal of Creativity in Mental Health, 9*, 292–392. 10.1080/15401383.2014.906874

Sileo, F. J., & Kopala, M. (1993). An A-B-C-D-E worksheet for promoting beneficence when considering ethical issues. *Counseling and Values, 37*(2), 89–95. 10.1002/j.2161-007X.1993.tb00800.x

Simon, R. M., & Graham, S. A. (2005). *Self-healing through visual and verbal art therapy.* Jessica Kingsley Publishers

Slayton, S. C., D'Archer, J., & Kaplan, F. (2010). Outcome studies on the efficacy of art therapy: A review of findings. *Art Therapy: Journal of the American Art Therapy Association, 27*(3), 108–119. 10.1080/07421656.2010.10129660

Sprigham, N. (2008). Through the eyes of the law: What is it about art that can harm people? *International Journal of Art Therapy, 13*(2), 65–73. 10.1080/17454 830802489141

Stone, C. B. (2009). *School counseling principles: Ethics and law* (2nd ed.). American School Counselor Association.

Sumner, W. G. (2008). Folkways: *A study of the sociological importance of usages, manners, customs, mores, and morals.* http://www.gutenberg.org/files/24253/24253-h/24253-h.htm (Original work published 1906)

Talwar, S. (2017). Ethics, law, and cultural competence in art therapy. *Art Therapy: Journal of the American Art Therapy Association, 34*(3), 102–105. 10.1 080/07421656.2017.1358026

Van Lith, T., & Voronin, L. (2016). Practicum learnings for counseling and art therapy students: The shared and the particular. *International Journal for the Advancement of Counseling, 38*(3), 177–193. 10.1007/s10447-016-9263-x

Vick, R. M. (2011). Ethics on exhibit. *Art Therapy: Journal of the American Art Therapy Association, 28*(4), 152–158. 10.1080/07421656.2011.622698

Warburton, N. (2013). *Philosophy: The basics* (5th ed.). Routledge. 10.4324/ 9781315817224

Ward v. Wilbanks. (2010). No. 09-CV-112 37, 2010 U.S. Dist. WL3026428 (E. D. Michigan, July 26, 2010).

Welfel, E. R. (2016). *Ethics in counseling and psychotherapy: Standards, research, and emerging issues* (6th ed.). Cengage.

Woody, R. H. (2013). *Legal self-defense for mental health practitioners.* Springer.

Zappa, A. (2017). Beyond erasure: The ethics of art therapy research with trans and gender-independent people. *Art Therapy: Journal of the American Art Therapy Association, 34*(3), 129–134. 10.1080/07421656.2017.1343074

2 Art Therapy Ethical Decision-Making Models[1]

Jessica M. Hauck and Thomson J. Ling

It is clear that ethical decision-making includes multiple components and must take into account multiple perspectives. As the field of art therapy continues to grow and diversify, the use of an approachable ethical decision-making model that is theoretically grounded, logical, culturally competent, and applicable to a wide scope of cases is of critical importance. The DO ART Model (Hauck & Ling, 2016) and the DO ART Directive Model (Hauck & Ling, 2020) were the first ethical decision-making models to be published for art therapists. The DO ART Model (Hauck & Ling, 2016) incorporates existing ethical literature in the field of art therapy (e.g., Hinz, 2011; Kapitan, 2011; Moon & Nolan, 2020), is appropriate for therapists at all levels, and can be used in a variety of situations. This model can be used by practitioners to reduce ambiguity and lead to overall improved ethical decision-making (Hauck & Ling, 2016).

2.1 The Importance of Including Art in Ethical Decision-Making

The benefits of art-making are substantial for both art therapy clients and art therapists (e.g., Bucciarelli, 2016; Deaver, 2011; Fish, 2012; Markin et al., 2013; Moon, 2001). From the start of the profession, art therapists have engaged in personal art-making for a variety of professional reasons (Fish, 2012; Deaver, 2011; Jackson et al., 2008; Markin et al., 2013; Moon, 2001). Some examples include response art for self-care (Fish, 2006; Jones, 1983; Moon & Nolan, 2020) and working through countertransference (Kielo, 1991; Wolf, 1985). More recently, art therapists have included art to enhance supervision (Deaver, 2011; Fish, 2008; Jackson et al., 2008), reflect on therapeutic abilities (Fish, 2012), and gain insight to deepen the therapeutic relationship (Fish, 2006; Kapitan, 2010). In short, there has been much literature indicating that art-making informed by tenets of art therapy can provide valuable insight into decision-making, and help externalize the thought process (Bucciarelli, 2016; Czamanski-Cohen, 2012; Potash & Ho, 2011; Thompson, 2009). Indeed, art-making has been recommended for art therapy graduate

DOI: 10.4324/9781003175124-2

students to enhance their training experience (Orkibi, 2012) as well as for practicing art therapists (Brown, 2008).

Given that art-making is central to the effective practice of art therapy and has numerous benefits for art therapists, it seems necessary to include directives in an ethical decision-making process. It has been noted that art therapists are adept in visual communication (Moon, 2001), thus including art in the ethical decision-making process allows art therapists to utilize their strengths. Additionally, art therapy is known to be beneficial in bringing automatic thoughts to conscious awareness (Naumburg, 1966) and in allowing for information to be understood in a new and meaningful way (Marshall, 2007), making it helpful in decision-making. Thus, adding art to the decision-making process may assist art therapists in more effective reflection that better honors the traditions and pillars valued by the field.

The use of a series of directives or assessments in art therapy is common as it may provide a clearer picture of a complex situation. Several art directives have been developed for managing trauma; for example, The Check art therapy protocol entails a neurobiological-based series of five directives (Hass-Cohen et al., 2014). With regard to assessments, the H-T-P (House-Tree-Person) is a series of three drawing directives used to assess cognitive and emotional functioning and interpersonal relationships (Buck, 1948). Similarly, the DDS (Diagnostic Drawing Series) is a well-known assessment for diagnosis that uses three directives (Cohen et al., 1988, 1994). Finally, the LECATA (Levick Emotional and Cognitive Art Therapy Assessment) uses a series of five directives grounded in Piagetian and Freudian theory to assess childhood development (Levick, 2009; Levick & Siegel, 2015). Indeed, employing a series of directives is an effective way to sort through complex situations with multifaceted circumstances.

Although some clinicians are adept at thinking through ethical dilemmas logically, art therapists possess strength in visual and non-logical communication. Since ethical dilemmas are inherently complicated by nature, a structured art activity can simplify the decision-making process by organizing the components in a clear and concise way.

2.2 The DO ART Model for Ethical Decision-Making

The DO ART ethical decision-making model is a guide that can be used to facilitate an art therapist in navigating ethical questions and circumstances in their practice (Hauck & Ling, 2016). This model includes six steps using a mnemonic that can be approached using logic as well as art visualization. In the model, art therapists are asked to first identify a situation where an ethical dilemma exists (D-Dilemma) and apply the relevant ethical principles and codes to the situation. Next, positive and negative effects on individuals are considered (O-Outcomes). In the third step, art therapists are instructed to consult the literature as well as supervisors and colleagues in order to clarify ambiguities in the dilemma (A-Assistance). Fourth, art therapists are asked to consider the risk and exposure to risk in the decision-making process (R-Responsibility). Finally, practitioners combine knowledge learned and factors considered in the other steps to decide on the most ethical course of action (T-Take Action). We believe that art therapists should utilize several theoretical perspectives when faced with a situation. Thus, the DO ART model is structured to consider utilitarianism, moral relativism, and deontological legalism in the second, third, and fourth steps respectively.

Each of these steps can be completed verbally as well as visually. Indeed, verbal analysis and visual analysis may play a reciprocal role in analyzing ethical dilemmas, and the DO ART Model includes a set of prescribed visualizations that art therapists can use to make solid ethical decisions and honors the traditions and pillars valued by the field. With each step of the model, art directives are given suggestions that may benefit clinicians as they undertake the decision-making process. We suggest organizing the directives in a manner that compiles all components of the DO ART model into a single stable and all-encompassing art piece. For example, a piece of paper that is folded into thirds, with art on both sides, may be utilized to depict all sections of the model (see Figure 2.1 for "one-sheet" example) and allowing for psychological containment (Malchiodi, 2011; Riley, 1999; Rubin, 2009; Ulman & Dachinger, 1996).

The completed art piece may also act as a transitional object to help bridge internal reality with the outside world (Heckwolf et al., 2014; Ulman and Dachinger, 1996). It should be noted that containment can also occur with individual art made in each step. This may be particularly beneficial if the step includes multiple or complicated facets; for example, some art therapists may visually represent this need for containment in a variety of ways, including containers or jars, boundary lines (concrete or diffused), snow globes, balloons, mandalas, or other visual depictions of natural or human-made barriers.

In the one-sheet example, we suggest beginning with the outside left flap because Western cultures typically follow a left to right progression in the organization of information. However, the placement can be arranged right to left for linguistic compatibility. In the following sections, we describe each step of this process. Examples in this manuscript will utilize 2D art; however, 3D art is also acceptable (in this situation, a photo may be taken and attached in the space designated for that visualization). It should also be noted that sections can be visually represented in any medium or format that speaks to the therapist; this can include a multitude of art styles and approaches, organized in a variety of ways. Some clinicians or situations may benefit from using the one-sheet approach, while others may create a comprehensive series of separate pieces or a single piece that evolves throughout the steps. Some clinicians

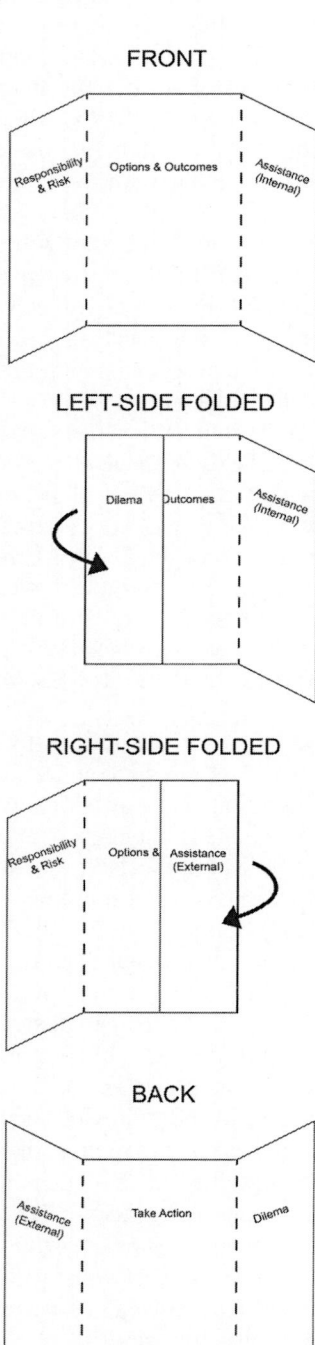

Figure 2.1 A "one-sheet" example of organizing art directives into a single stable and all-encompassing art piece.

may also choose to create other artwork, or photographs, to visually process the experience as a whole.

2.2.1 D-Dilemma

The identification of the ethical dilemma in an art therapy situation is the first step of the DO ART model and provides a clear reason for the application of the model. In many art therapy situations, several principles and/or codes may be applicable and may suggest different ethical behaviors. An ethical dilemma is defined as a situation where ethical principles and/or codes suggest different courses of action, meaning that an art therapist would not be able to abide by all applicable principles and codes. In these situations, the most ethical course of action requires a thorough analysis of the possible courses of actions, the weighing of various courses of action, and a conscious decision to engage in a course of action that may abide by some ethical principles and codes but not others. Another way to think about this is that an ethical dilemma exists where principles and codes are in opposition to one another.

The *Ethical Principles for Art Therapists* describe aspirational ethical principles for art therapists (American Art Therapy Association, 2013). In some situations, these principles provide clarity in an ethical situation. For example, American Art Therapy Association (2013) principle 2.2 clearly states that art therapists provide clients with information about the limits to confidentiality. However, in other cases, the ethical course of action is less clear. For example, American Art Therapy Association (2013) principle 5.2 indicates the importance of "proper safeguards" in exhibition but leaves it up to the art therapist to define a "proper safeguard". Similarly, American Art Therapy Association (2013) principle 14.4 suggests that art therapists involve clients appropriately in the process of termination; this can result in disagreement as to the "appropriate" amount of client involvement. Similar challenges exist with the Art Therapy Credentials Board Code of Ethics, Conduct, and Disciplinary Procedures (Art Therapy Credentials Board, 2021). To better understand this idea, Behnke (2006) describes ethical guidelines using the metaphor of a stoplight. In this metaphor, the specific principles and codes can be seen as communicating prohibited behavior via a red light, permitted behavior via a green light, and behavior where caution is suggested as a yellow light (Behnke, 2006).

In order to identify an ethical dilemma, it is recommended art therapists start by identifying the possible courses of action moving forward (i.e., options) and then thoroughly reviewing the various ethical principles or codes that might apply to that course of action. These may include the ethical principles for art therapists (American Art Therapy Association, 2013); the code of ethics, conduct, and disciplinary procedures (Art Therapy Credentials Board, 2021); the ethical guidelines for other professional organizations; or institutional guidelines. With each option, ethical principles may either support or discourage an option. While commonly ethical dilemmas will result in considering two options, this is not always the case and this model may be used to consider three or more options if the situation necessitates.

As art therapists consider options, three potential types of options may emerge. First, an option may exist where all applicable principles are supporting that option. In this situation, no ethical dilemma exists and there is no need to apply an ethical decision-making model. Second, an option may exist where no principles support the course of action. In this situation, this option should not be considered. Finally, an option may exist such that art therapists would be abiding by some of the ethical principles but not others. This third category is most common to art therapy ethical situations and typically multiple options fit under this category. Thus, an ethical dilemma exists when there are no options that allow the therapist to abide by all applicable principles.

A common misconception is that ethical decision-making is the correction of previous behaviors or actions that violate ethical codes. While primary prevention is important in ethical practice, once violations have occurred, the focus of decision-making switches the remediation (Welfel, 2016). Practitioners often find it challenging to separate out previous ethics code violations from remediating actions moving forward (Welfel, 2016). It may be helpful for art therapists to only consider previous behaviors or actions in the context of how they may affect behaviors moving forward. For example, if an art therapist did not realize a burnt-out light bulb was resulting in inadequate lighting for a client, their focus would be on ensuring there is adequate lighting for subsequent sessions since it would not be possible to prevent violations that have already occurred (i.e., the inadequate lighting in prior sessions). Once an ethical dilemma is identified, it becomes clear that the rest of the DO ART model is needed to determine which course of action is most ethical given that it is impossible to adhere to all relevant ethical principles.

Visually, the dilemma stage can be depicted in many ways. For example, this information could be represented using continuum lines to describe the ethical implications of identified codes. If using the one-sheet example, these lines could be placed on the outside left flap. However, art therapists are not limited to this visualization or organization. For example, an art therapist could use an abstract image to process the dilemma. In addition, an infographic-style art piece visually representing the codes and principles might be utilized. Other examples include an image that represents each considered option. In short, there are many ways an art therapist could visually represent the dilemma as part of the ethical decision-making process.

2.2.2 O-Outcomes

The second step in the DO ART model is to examine the positive and negative outcomes for each option. Art therapists examine options independently to determine all likely consequences. To do this, it is important to first identify all constituents or stakeholders who would likely be affected by the option selected. This is in alignment with the fidelity principle identified in the preamble of the Ethical Principles of Art Therapists (American Art Therapy Association, 2013). Although stakeholders always include the client and art therapist, other constituents may include but are not limited to: other clients of the art therapists, family members, colleagues, and the communities the art therapists work with. By identifying all relevant constituents the art therapist is able to consider the totality of the situation as opposed to only considering the client.

After identifying relevant constituents, the art therapist should go on to consider how each of these constituents is affected by the various options. A question an art therapist should ask is "does this constituent experience any desirable outcomes by the selection of this option?" Similarly, the art therapist should also ask "does this constituent suffer any undesirable consequences as a result of this option?" Art therapists can think of this step as determining the advantages and disadvantages of each option for all relevant parties.

The outcomes step can be depicted using several visualizations. For example, some visual methods might include: (1) a libra scale that represents the weighing of options, (2) the two lenses on a pair of glasses might represent the different viewpoints that each option presents, (3) individual drawings that represent each option, or (4) another way of visually compartmentalizing the options. If using the one-sheet example, depicted in Figure 2.1, clinicians should open the paper to the inside middle section and begin by representing these options in a visual or text-based format. Again, art therapists can use a multitude of art directives here. For example, some clinicians may want to represent this step with an abstract piece depicting the options, while others may choose to fold/divide their piece in half and create two separate images. Further, the art therapist may focus on the emotional impact of each outcome beyond the outcomes themselves.

2.2.3 A-Assistance

In any ethical dilemma, art therapists should seek assistance to ensure they are acting in alignment with other art therapists who are in similar circumstances as well as stay up to date with industry-standard practices. Indeed, the *Ethical Principles for Art Therapists* (American Art Therapy Association, 2013), the *Art Therapy Credentials Board Code of Ethics, Conduct, and Professional Practice* (Art Therapy Credentials Board, 2021), and the *Art Therapy Multicultural/Diversity Competencies* (American Art Therapy Association, 2011) encourages consultation with others. In addition, art therapists should also consider relevant art therapy literature and ethics literature to expand the scope of assistance available. It should be noted that there is a difference between receiving assistance and receiving a decision from a consultant. Art therapists should avoid the latter as it moves the responsibility for the decision away from the art therapist while not necessarily moving the liability for the decision to a consultant. In other words, while it is important to consider the assistance received from others, art therapists should always combine this assistance with the other steps of the DO ART model.

In the assistance step, art therapists should start by considering appropriate consultation questions. Starting with the framework developed by Behnke (2014), consultation questions can be legal questions, ethical questions, clinical questions, or risk management questions. An additional question about art materials may also be appropriate because art therapy may raise ethical concerns specific to art materials. Legal questions consider how laws and regulations may apply to a situation. Ethical questions involve the interpretation of the ethical principles that apply. Clinical questions involve how actions may affect the best interests of the client in the context of their culture. Risk management questions consider exposure to liability. Art material questions consider the appropriateness and potential impact of specific materials. Behnke (2014) suggests that understanding whether a question is legal, ethical, clinical, or risk management informs whom the art therapist should consult. Legal questions may involve an attorney, ethical questions may involve the art therapy ethics board, clinical questions may involve a supervisor, risk-management questions may involve a liability insurance company, and art material questions may involve a colleague or supervisor.

In addition, art therapists should also consult relevant laws, regulations, and current literature in an ethical dilemma. Because laws, regulations, and best practices may change over time, it is important for art therapists to be familiar with the prevailing thought on a situation. Art therapists should ensure that they are examining current literature, including journal articles concerning related topics, pertinent cultural considerations, previous ethics cases, and relevant laws/regulations in their jurisdiction. Once these sources are identified, an art therapist can consider how information from each source supports or does not support the various options.

There are various methods that can be used to visually represent this process. During the assistance stage, clinicians examine information that is gathered from external sources (i.e., consultants and literature). However, recognizing that information acquired from outside sources is also processed internally, it is important to represent both parts of this process. The assistance step is organized in this way to demonstrate the complex yet necessary interplay between gathering external information and processing that information internally. To this end, if the one-sheet example is being used, clinicians should utilize both the front and back sides of the right flap to depict this stage. The outside part of the right flap represents external sources and art therapists should begin by investigating relevant research and consulting with knowledgeable and experienced professionals. This information should then be identified in a way that provides a clear yet succinct overview during which different colors, art materials, and arrangements may be considered. Once all of the relevant information has been identified this information should be integrated with an art visualization that illustrates the internal processes on the inside right flap.

In creating these art representations there is an opportunity to consider how each lends support for or discourages each option. For example, an art therapist could create a set of images that represent different sources of assistance, a visual depiction of how assistance is combined to create a final product, or an image that showcases some level of tension that is felt between different assistance sources. In our experience, art therapists can occasionally feel overwhelmed by the sheer number of assistance sources considered and this is where artwork with themes of containment might be particularly beneficial, though certainly not required.

2.2.4 R-Responsibility/Risk

In the responsibility or risk step, art therapists revisit the various stake-holders identified in the outcome step (e.g., client, other clients, and their agency). It is likely that for each of these stakeholders, the art therapist has some responsibility and their actions may expose them to risk. Examining responsibilities and risks by stakeholders accounts for the possibility that actions may simultaneously increase and decrease exposure to liability. For example, while an option may allow the art therapist to fulfill their responsibilities for one client, it may simultaneously cause the art therapist to increase their exposure to risk with a different client.

An additional benefit of this step is that an art therapist can also identify strategies to mitigate risk. For example, an art therapist might determine that revisiting the informed consent process would be helpful in a situation to minimize risk exposure with a client.

To visually represent and externally organize this information, art therapists have several different options. If using the one-sheet example an art directive for this stage can be completed on the inside left flap (if entirely unfolded). Art therapists may illustrate the balance between taking on risks and managing various responsibilities in several ways. Art therapists might utilize the Draw-a-Person-in-the-Rain directive that typically assesses stress and coping (Willis et al., 2010; Verinis et al., 1974). Applied to ethical decision-making, this assessment is modified so that risk is represented by the rain and management of responsibility is represented by protection from the rain. Another example of a balance-focused directive could be a drawing of a tree, with the root design symbolizing the depth of responsibility an art therapist holds in this situation, while the branches depict the amount of risk that may be present. The roots of responsibility would indicate the foundation and ground that is necessary in all art therapy practice whereas branches would indicate how risk, if managed appropriately, can be beneficial to certain relevant parties. Likewise, unexamined risk can negatively impact the balance and topple the tree. As with the outcome step, art therapists may find it helpful to also visualize the emotions connected with balancing risk and responsibility. Some other examples of visually representing risk and responsibility include artwork that illustrates holding the weight of a decision, or creating a boundary that protects an art therapist from exposure to risk.

2.2.5 T-Take Action

The final step of the DO ART model is to take action and often the appropriate ethical decision emerges as a result of the thoughtful and informed analysis of the complex factors in the previous steps. Specifically, the art therapist should be able to identify the most ethical and/or the least unethical option among those considered. This choice can be further confirmed by revisiting any completed art directives from previous steps and considering them in their totality.

Visually this can be depicted in several ways. If utilizing the one-sheet example, art therapists should flip the handout over completely and use the back middle section to illustrate the last step of their decision-making process, and emphasize what it looks like to move forward with the dilemma resolved. One art therapy directive that may be utilized is the Bridge Drawing which is typically used to assess the process and impact of change, and commitment to goals (Darewych, 2014; Hays & Lyons, 1981). Applied to ethical decision-making it can depict where they are on their journey towards making and implementing a course of action. Similarly, a road drawing has traditionally been used to uncover intentions for the future and to assess recovery and capacity for change (Hanes, 1995, 2008, 2017), but may be adapted to represent the path practitioners must take to resolve the dilemma with potential barriers, roadblocks, and detours included. Other examples may include an image that depicts the resolution of the dilemma, or the ethical decision-making process as a journey. Art therapists may also choose to create just one piece of artwork over the course of the DO ART model, which emerges as they progress through the steps; with each step, additional modifications are made to the piece resulting in a finalized product during the final stage. Regardless of the visual representation selected this step allows for the documentation and justification of actions an art therapist takes.

2.3 Summary

Overall, The DO ART model both supports a selected course of action and serves as a tool to document the thought process used to reach that decision in a method that speaks to the unique strengths of art therapists. Further, the DO ART model allows for effective communication of a decision-making process both verbally and visually should the selected action ever be questioned. Because good ethical decision-making requires assessing the full impact of any actions taken, the DO ART model gives art therapists the tools to make an ethically informed decision that is defensible and in alignment with best practices.

Note

1 This book is derived in part from two articles published in Art Therapy: Journal of the American Art Therapy Association (2013, 2020) copyright American Art Therapy Association, available online: http://www.tandfonline.com/10.1080/ 07421656.2016.1231544; http://www.tandfonline.com/10.1080/07421656.2019.1 667669

References

American Art Therapy Association. (2011). *Art therapy multicultural/diversity competencies.* https://arttherapy.org/wp-content/uploads/2017/06/Multicultural-Competencies.pdf

American Art Therapy Association. (2013). *Ethical principles for art therapists.* https://arttherapy.org/wp-content/uploads/2017/06/Ethical-Principles-for-Art-Therapists.pdf

Art Therapy Credentials Board. (2021). *Code of ethics, conduct, and disciplinary procedures.* https://www.atcb.org/wp-content/uploads/2020/07/ATCB-Code-of-Ethics-Conduct-DisciplinaryProcedures.pdf

Behnke, S. H. (2006). Beyond mere compliance: Three metaphors to teach the APA ethics code. *Monitor on Psychology, 37*(11), 54. http://www.apa.org/monitor/dec06/ethics.aspx

Behnke, S. H. (2014). What kind of issue is it? A "four-bin" approach to ethics consultation is helpful in practical settings. *Monitor on Psychology, 45*(2), 62. http://www.apa.org/monitor/2014/02/issue.aspx

Brown, C. (2008). The importance of making art for the creative arts therapist: An artistic inquiry. *Arts in Psychotherapy, 35*(3), 201–208. 10.1016/j.aip.2008.04.002

Bucciarelli, A. (2016). Art therapy: A transdisciplinary approach. *Art Therapy: Journal of the American Art Therapy Association, 33*(3), 151–155. 10.1080/07421656.2016.1199246

Buck, J. N. (1948). The H-T-P test. *Journal of Clinical Psychology, 4*(2), 151–159. 10.1002/1097-4679(194804)4:2<151::AID-JCLP2270040203>3.0.CO;2-O

Cohen, B., Hammer, J., & Singer, S. (1988). The diagnostic drawing series: A systematic approach to art therapy evaluation and research. *The Arts in Psychotherapy, 15,* 11–21. 10.1016/0197-4556(88)90048-2

Cohen, B. M., Mills, A., & Kijak, A. K. (1994). An introduction to the diagnostic drawing series: A standardized tool for diagnostic and clinical use. *Art Therapy: Journal of the American Art Therapy Association, 11*(2), 105–110. 10.1 080/07421656.1994.10759060

Czamanski-Cohen, J. (2012). The use of art in the medical decision-making process of oncology patients. *Art Therapy: Journal of the American Art Therapy Association, 29*(2), 60–67 10.1080/07421656.2012.680049

Darewych, O. H. (2014). *The bridge drawing with path art-based assessment: Measuring meaningful life pathways in higher education students* (Doctoral dissertation). Lesley University.

Deaver, S. P. (2011). Research ethics: Institutional review board oversight of art therapy research. *Art Therapy: Journal of the American Art Therapy Association, 28*(4), 171–176. 10.1080/07421656.2011.622685

Fish, B. J. (2006). *Image-based narrative inquiry of response art in art therapy* (Doctoral dissertation). Retrieved from ProQuest Dissertations and Thesis database. (UMI No. 3228081)

Fish, B. J. (2008). Formative evaluation research of art-based supervision in art therapy training. *Art Therapy: Journal of the American Art Therapy Association, 25*(2): 70–77. 10.1080/07421656.2008.10129410

Fish, B. J. (2012). Response art: The art of the art therapist. *Art Therapy: Journal of the American Art Therapy Association, 29*(3), 138–143. 10.1080/07421656. 2012.701594

Hanes, M. (2017). Road to recovery: Road drawings in a gender-specific residential substance use treatment center. *Art Therapy: Journal of the American Art Therapy Association, 34*(4), 201–208. 10.1080/07421656.2017.1394124

Hanes, M. J. (1995). Utilizing road drawings as a therapeutic metaphor in art therapy. *American Journal of Art Therapy, 34,* 19–19.

Hanes, M. J. (2008). Signs of suicide: Using road drawings with inmates on suicide observation at a county jail. *Art Therapy: Journal of the American Art Therapy Association, 25*(2), 78–84. 10.1080/07421656.2008.10129418

Hass-Cohen, N., Clyde Findlay, J., Carr, R., & Vanderlan, J. (2014). "Check, change what you need to change and/or keep what you want": An art therapy neurobiological-based trauma protocol. *Art Therapy: Journal of the American Art Therapy Association, 31*(2), 69–78. 10.1080/07421656.2014.903825

Hauck, J., & Ling, T. (2016). The DO ART model: An ethical decision-making model applicable to art therapy. *Art Therapy: Journal of the American Art Therapy Association, 33*(4), 203–208. 10.1080/07421656.2016.1231544

Hauck, J. M., & Ling, T. J. (2020). Applying art therapy directives to ethical decision-making. *Art Therapy: Journal of the American Art Therapy Association. 37*(1), 34–41. 10.1080/07421656.2019.1667669

Hays, R. E., & Lyons, S. J. (1981). The bridge drawing: A projective technique for assessment in art therapy. *The Arts in Psychotherapy, 8,* 207–217. 10.1016/0197-4556(81)90033-2

Heckwolf, J. I., Bergland, M. C., & Mouratidis, M. (2014). Coordinating principles of art therapy and DBT. *The Arts in Psychotherapy*, *41*(4), 329–335. 10.1016/j.aip.2014.03.006

Hinz, L.D. (2011). Embracing excellence: A positive approach to ethical decision making. *Art Therapy: Journal of the American Art Therapy Association*, *28*(4). 185–188. 10.1080/07421656.2011.622693

Jackson, S., Muro, J., Lee, Y., & DeOrnellas, K. (2008). The sacred circle: Using mandalas in counselor supervision. *Journal of Creativity in Mental Health*, *3*, 201–211. 10.1080/15401380802369164

Jones, D. L. (1983). An art therapist's personal record. *Art Therapy: Journal of the American Art Therapy Association*, *1*(1): 22–25. 10.1080/07421656.1983.10758734

Kapitan, L. (2010). *Introduction to art therapy research*. Taylor & Francis Group.

Kapitan, L. (2011). "But is it ethical?" Articulating an art therapy ethos. *Art Therapy: Journal of the American Art Therapy Association*, *28*(4), 150–151. 10.1080/07421656.2011.624930

Kielo, J. B. (1991). Art therapists' countertransference and post-session therapy imagery. *Art Therapy: Journal of the American Art Therapy Association*, *8*(2): 14–19. 10.1080/07421656.1991.10758923

Levick, M. F. (2009). *Levick emotional and cognitive art therapy assessment: A normative study*. AuthorHouse.

Levick, M. F., & Siegel, C. A. (2015). The Levick emotional and cognitive art therapy assessment (LECATA). In D. E. Gussak, & M. L. Rosal (Eds.), *The Wiley Handbook of Art Therapy* (pp. 534–549). Wiley-Blackwell.

Malchiodi, C. A. (Ed.). (2011). *Handbook of art therapy*. Guilford Press.

Markin, R. D., McCarthy, K. S., & Barber, J. P. (2013). Transference, countertransference, emotional expression, and session quality over the course of supportive expressive therapy: The rater's perspective. *Psychotherapy Research*, *23*, 152–168. 10.1080/10503307/2012.747013

Marshall, J. (2007). Image as insight: Visual images in practice-based research. *Studies in Art Education*, *49*(1), 23–41. 10.1080/00393541.2007.11518722

Moon, C. (2001). *Studio art therapy: Cultivating the artist identity in the art therapist*. Jessica Kingsley Publishers.

Moon, B. L., & Nolan, E. G. (2020). *Ethical issues in art therapy* (4th ed.). Charles C. Thomas.

Naumburg, M. (1966). *Dynamically oriented art therapy: Its principles and practices, illustrated with three case studies*. Grune & Stratton.

Orkibi, H. (2012). Students' artistic experience before and during graduate training. *The Arts In Psychotherapy*, *39*(5), 428–435. 10.1016/j.aip.2012.06.007

Potash, J., & Ho, R. T. (2011). Drawing involves caring: Fostering relationship building through art therapy for social change. *Art Therapy: Journal of the American Art Therapy Association*, *28*(2), 74–81. 10.1080/07421656.2011.578040

Riley, S. (1999). *Contemporary art therapy with adolescents*. Jessica Kingsley Publishers.

Rubin, J. A. (2009). *Introduction to art therapy: Sources & resources*. Routledge.

Thompson, G. (2009). Artistic sensibility in the studio and gallery model: Revisiting process and product. *Art Therapy: Journal of the American Art Therapy Association*, *26*(4), 159–166. 10.1080/07421656.2009.10129609

Ulman, E., & Dachinger, P. (1996). *Art therapy in theory & practice*. Magnolia Street Publishers.

Verinis, J. S., Lichtenberg, E. F., & Henrich, L. (1974). The Draw-a-Person-in-the-Rain technique: Its relationship to diagnostic category and other personality indicators. *Journal of Clinical Psychology, 30*(3), 407–414. 10.1002/1097-4679(197407)30:3<407::AID-JCLP2270300358>3.0.CO;2-6

Welfel, E. R. (2016). *Ethics in counseling and psychotherapy: Standards, research, and emerging issues* (6th ed.). Cengage.

Willis, L. R., Joy, S. P., & Kaiser, D. H. (2010). Draw-a-Person-in-the-Rain as an assessment of stress and coping resources. *The Arts in Psychotherapy, 37*(3), 233–239. 10.1016/j.aip.2010.04.009

Wolf, R. (1985). Image induction in the countertransference: A revision of the totalistic view. *Art Therapy: Journal of the American Art Therapy Association, 2*(3), 120–133.

3 Artist, Therapist, Art Therapist or Something Else: Navigating Multiple Professional Identities

Laura Holland and Jenna Pattison

Art therapists have long debated over their professional identities, with many attaining multiple clinical licenses and identifying as artists as well as art therapists. Having multiple professional identities is a common occurrence, but even more so with art therapists. Art therapists often define themselves as a combination between artists, art therapists, teachers, advocates, and counselors. Indeed, research has identified that one of the challenges art therapists in training face is seeing how art therapy and other creative modalities intersect with mental health counseling (e.g., Degges-White & Davis, 2017; McNiff, 2009; Van Lith & Voronin, 2016). Likewise, the question of how using creativity in counseling intersects with art therapy has been examined (Rosen & Atkins, 2014). Due to the variety of roles art therapists can fill, and the variety of other professions they may work within treatment teams, they may experience a tension between their multiple professional identities and roles. The necessity of multiple professional identities is further evident by the fact that a majority of states do not provide a clear path for licensure as an art therapist. Only five states provide art therapy-specific licenses (Kentucky, Maryland, Mississippi, New Jersey, and New Mexico) and five additional states allow for art therapists to gain licensure under related areas (New York, Pennsylvania, Texas, Utah, and Washington) (Rastogi, 2017). This chapter will focus on the ethical challenges that are present in navigating multiple professional identities.

3.1 The Case of Veronica

Veronica, an art therapist and mental health counselor, recently started working at an adolescent psychiatric residential facility. Veronica is the only art therapist on staff and the only dual licensed clinician at her site. There has never been an art therapist at this location before, and Veronica is excited to introduce art therapy as a treatment modality to the facility.

Veronica's responsibilities include co-leading a weekly group for the youth with her colleague Eric, a mental health counselor. Veronica and Eric have a good working relationship and have really enjoyed co-leading the group. Eric recently shared with Veronica that he is excited about the

DOI: 10.4324/9781003175124-3

art therapy interventions Veronica is bringing to the facility. He stated that as he has looked for new ways to engage in self-care to cope with work stress, he found an art therapy mandala coloring book online. He explained that coloring the mandalas "helped so much to relax" when he got home from work. Eric tells Veronica he feels inspired by the work he has seen her do with the youth and the new ideas she brings to the group. Veronica and Eric take turns planning the topics and facilitating the activities for the group each week. This arrangement has worked well for them so far because it allows each of them to bring their own expertise to the group. This week was Eric's turn and after Eric opens the group and completes the check-in, he starts presenting the activity. He excitedly states that the group will be doing art therapy today. He discloses how art therapy has worked well for him recently to reduce stress and he wants to teach it to the group so that they can utilize it as a coping skill. Eric goes on to say that they will be coloring their own mandalas, and that he will provide extra copies for the youth to use in their free time. Before Veronica has a chance to say anything, Amy, a group member who is usually resistant and guarded, explains "I saw art therapy mandala coloring books online also! I'm so excited to try this, I've been debating asking my parents to buy me some of them for my birthday." This prompts the group members to discuss the art therapy adult coloring books they have seen or their friends have had. Some group members disclose that they own art therapy coloring books and declare how much these books have helped. For example, one group member, Christopher, says "I do my own art therapy all the time when I do little doodles to express my feelings!" The group goes well, and all the group members end up participating, leaving the group in a brighter mood and engaging with each other more than Eric or Veronica have seen in the past.

After the group session, Eric mentions how successful the mandala group session was to Elizabeth, the Clinical Director. The clinical director, who is also a mental health counselor, praises Eric for his idea and expresses interest in having Eric share the mandala activities with other counselors in the residential facility.

Veronica is stunned that Eric would choose to facilitate an art therapy activity, and that their clinical director requested Eric to share art therapy activities with other counselors in the facility. This is particularly unusual because in the past, the clinical director has been hesitant to bring Veronica on board to do more art therapy, saying that other counselors "do plenty of arts and crafts" with the youth in creative expression groups.

3.2 Analysis of Case

In the case of Veronica and Eric, Veronica must decide if using the mandala coloring pages qualifies as art therapy and if she should confront

Eric practicing outside his scope. Veronica needs to decide if confronting Eric will help protect their clients and other clinicians at the site from practicing outside of their scope. Veronica must also decide if she should confront her clinical director, taking into consideration that she could lose her position if she does since she is a new addition to the team.

3.2.1 D-Dilemma

In this case, Veronica, an art therapist and mental health counselor, and Eric, a mental health counselor, co-facilitate a group at a youth psychiatric residential facility. Eric used what he called an art therapy directive with the group and the youth responded very well to it. Now, the clinical director wants Eric to share the directive with the other counselors on site.

As a result, Veronica has two options. Option one is that Veronica decides the directive is art therapy and that she should confront Eric and the clinical director to prevent other mental health counselors from using the mandala activity. She would do this to ensure clients are protected from a therapist practicing outside their scope. Veronica would educate the staff and director about art therapy to help protect and advocate for the field. However, as a new clinician, Veronica is concerned about going against the clinical director, alienating other clinicians, and her job security.

Option two is that Veronica, taking the perspective of a mental health counselor, decides the coloring pages are not art therapy and therefore does not need to confront Eric or the director. She would be able to continue to co-facilitate the group with Eric, and their clients would likely continue to benefit, In this option, Veronica would not only be able to maintain her professional relationships and continue to work with her clients, but she would be allowing other clinicians and clients to explore utilizing art as a coping skill, which mental health counselors occasionally do. However, she is concerned that she would not be advocating for art therapy, would be misleading clients about what art therapy is, and promoting other clinicians to practice outside their scope.

In Figure 3.1, Veronica utilizes art to work through the dilemma. She uses stacks to books to represent each option, with each book representing a code that supports the options. This helps her to realize she has an ethical dilemma on her hands that requires both research and careful consideration.

3.2.1.1 Option One: Principles Supporting Option One

Option one, which would be deciding the directive was art therapy and confronting Eric and the clinical director, is supported by several principles. Veronica would be upholding code 1.1.1 in which art therapists respect the rights and welfare of their clients and make reasonable efforts

Figure 3.1 Two stacks of books of equal sizes illustrating the Dilemma stage.

to ensure art therapy is used appropriately (Art Therapy Credentials Board [ATCB], 2021). Principle 1.7 is also crucial in this case, as Veronica would use supervision to discuss how to appropriately confront the other clinicians (American Art Therapy Association [AATA], 2013). She would also be upholding principle 8.3 in which art therapists take reasonable steps to ensure that others do not present themselves as competent to perform professional services which are beyond their scope (American Art Therapy Association, 2013). She would also be upholding principle 10.1 to adhere to the ethical principles of AATA, of which she is a member (American Art Therapy Association, 2013). Lastly, she would be upholding 10.8 by preventing the misuse of art therapy in an organization that she is a part of (American Art Therapy Association, 2013). Veronica would also be abiding by principle I.2.a (American Counseling Association [ACA], 2014) that states that if a counselor has a reason to believe another counselor is committing an ethics violation, they should attempt to resolve it informally with the counselor.

3.2.1.2 Option One: Codes and Principles Discouraging Option One

Although there are many principles supporting option one, there are others that discourage it. In upholding principle 1.1 (American Art Therapy Association, 2013) and code 1.1.4 (ATCB, 2021), she would be respecting the rights of her clients to make their own decisions in what coping skills they choose to take from the group. As a mental health counselor, there are no codes or principles that would prohibit the use of a mandala as an intervention. Principle 1.5 is also crucial in that if she confronts Eric and it does not go well, she may not be able to keep her personal feelings from preventing her from performing her duties to the group (American Art Therapy Association, 2013). Principle 6.4 states that art therapists must cooperate with other professionals to serve the clients, and by not confronting Eric she would uphold this principle due to the fact that the directive went very well with the group (American Art Therapy Association, 2013). She would also be ensuring she follows code 1.1.7 that states art therapists must not abandon their clients, as she believes there is a chance she may lose her position if the confrontation with the clinical director does not go well (ATCB, 2021). Code 1.1.12 states that art therapists must not make improper ethical complaints against their colleagues, and by not confronting Eric and potentially re-porting him when she is unsure if the directive was art therapy, Veronica would be upholding this principle (ATCB, 2021). She would also be advancing the use of art therapy in code 1.5.1 if she allowed other clin-icians at the site to utilize the directive (ATCB, 2021). Lastly, code 2.3.10 states that art therapists shall be aware of and take into account the practices of other professions and cooperate with them (ATCB, 2021). By not confronting the director and other clinicians, Veronica, as an art therapist, would be respecting that other treatment modalities (e.g., mental health counselors) may use creativity, just in a different way than art therapists do.

3.2.1.3 Option Two: Principles Supporting Option Two

Option two, which is to not confront Eric or her director due to her decision that the directive is not art therapy, is supported by several principles. Principle 1.1 (American Art Therapy Association, 2013) and code 1.1.4 (ATCB, 2021) state that art therapists respect the rights of their clients to make decisions. By not confronting Eric, Veronica would be in alignment with her responsibility as a mental health counselor and trusting her clients to make the decision to utilize what works for them from their groups. It is also stated in principle 6.4 that art therapists will cooperate with other professionals (e.g., mental health counselors), which Veronica and Eric have done well so far and can continue to do if there is no confrontation (American Art Therapy Association, 2013). Specifically, clients will benefit because effective group treatment can continue. Since she is also debating if the directive is even art therapy, it may be unethical for her to make a claim against Eric practicing outside his scope as evi-denced by code1.1.12 (ATCB, 2021). Veronica is also potentially re-specting the rights of her colleague to practice as he sees fit as stated in code 1.5.1 (ATCB, 2021). Lastly, code 2.3.10 states that art therapists should take into account the practices of other professions and cooperate with them, and many other therapists utilize creativity in their practice (ATCB, 2021).

3.2.1.4 Option Two: Codes and Principles Discouraging Option Two

Despite many principles that encourage option two, there are many that also discourage it. Code 1.1.1 states that art therapists shall ensure that their services are being used appropriately, and by not speaking up Veronica, in her art therapist role, maybe encouraging other clinicians (e.g., mental health counselors) to misuse art therapy (ATCB, 2021). Principle 1.7 states that art therapists seek supervision when encountering issues, and if she does not speak up or utilize supervision to work through this problem, then she is not upholding this principle (American Art Therapy Association, 2013). It is also crucial that principles 8.3 and 8.6 be considered as they state that art therapists take reasonable steps to ensure supervisees do not practice beyond their training and when training non-art therapists one must take precautions to ensure trainees understand that is different from a formal education in art therapy (American Art Therapy Association, 2013). Though Veronica is not supervising or training Eric, she should make it clear to him that she is not teaching him art therapy and even though he co-facilitates the group with her, it may not make it appropriate for him to utilize art therapy. By not speaking up Veronica may also be violating principle 10.1 which states she must ad-here to the ethical principles of her art therapy professional organization (American Art Therapy Association, 2013), but not her mental health counseling professional association. Lastly, principle 10.8 states that an art therapist must prevent the misuse of art therapy by an institution they are a part of (American Art Therapy Association, 2013). Veronica would also be violating principle I.2.a (American Counseling Association, 2014) that states that if a counselor has a reason to believe another counselor is committing an ethics violation, they should attempt to resolve it in-formally with the counselor.

3.2.2 O-Outcome

Although Veronica is making a simple choice of considering whether or not to confront Eric about his directive, there are many other people that may be affected by the outcome of this scenario. In both Options one and two, the possible constituents or stakeholders would be Veronica, Eric, the clinical director, the clients in the group, other therapists in their residential facility, as well as the other clients at the residential facility.

The weighing of these options is further expressed in Figure 3.2. Through art, Veronica may review the two options that she has and

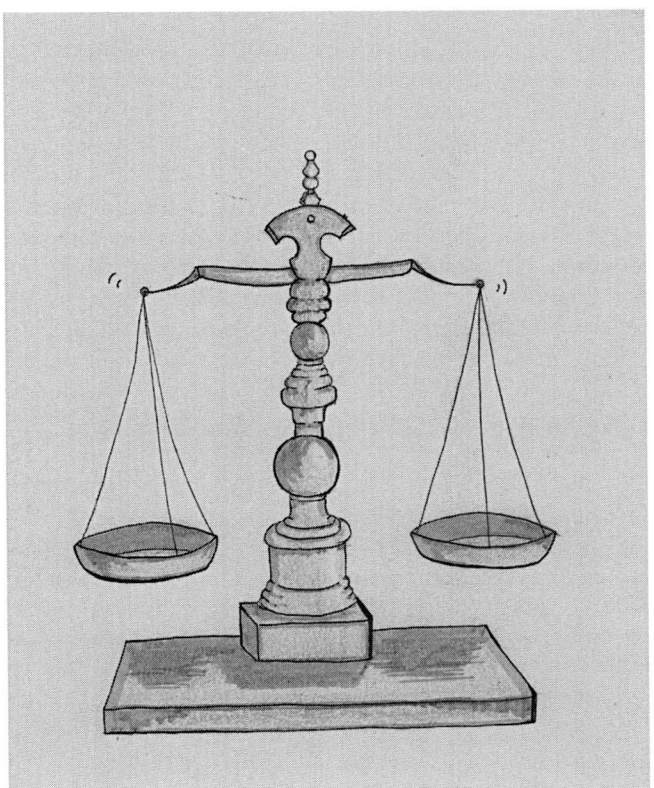

Figure 3.2 A balanced but shaky libra scale depicting the difficulty in weighing options.

consider how heavy the outcomes of each would be. The scales are balanced but are shaky, representing the ease in which one option might tip the scale in either direction.

3.2.2.1 Option One

In Option One, Veronica herself would be affected in a positive way. Veronica would be fulfilling her obligation as an art therapist to advocate for her field and prevent others from misusing or misinterpreting art therapy. On the other hand, confronting Eric may be received poorly, leading Veronica to become ostracized by her coworkers and director (especially those that share her mental health counselor identity), which would be distressing. Even more so, Veronica might not be fulfilling her role as a counselor if she is deemed unable to work together with her peers effectively. Eric would be negatively affected by this option because if he is seen as practicing outside of his scope of practice, his position as a mental health counselor may be in jeopardy or is at risk of being reprimanded by the clinical director. The clinical director, Elizabeth, would benefit from this result. While Elizabeth may be surprised by Veronica addressing her concerns, overall, the clinical director would be at less risk of her facility facing unethical treatment practices and possible malpractice issues later. In this option, Veronica and Eric's group members might be negatively affected depending on how Eric responds to Veronica's confrontation. If well-received, Veronica and Eric might be able to discuss art therapy more in-depth with the youth in their group and give them a better understanding of what art therapy looks like, thus benefiting them. If the confrontation is not well received, the pair's clients may be affected negatively if Veronica and Eric are separated or choose not to work together moving forward due to the confrontation. The adolescents in their group are at high risk as it is and any possible act perceived as abandonment after such positive results may cause clients distress or harm. The response from other clinicians and staff in the facility can vary from person to person. Some staff members might feel relieved that Veronica prevented them from misusing art therapy or practicing outside of their scope. Other staff members might be negatively affected due to discomfort or disagreement with Veronica's choice. Staff might not feel that what Eric did was wrong or do not see his directive as art therapy as they have also used art as a tool within their own practices. Other clients in the residential facility have a chance of being affected positively through this option by not being exposed to misused art therapy practices from inexperienced clinicians.

3.2.2.2 Option Two

In Option Two, Veronica would benefit positively to a certain extent. Veronica would remain in good standing with both Eric and the rest of the residential facility staff by not confronting Eric. While this would bring her temporary peace, Veronica may be negatively affected long-term if Eric continues to use what she perceives as art therapy and spreads this practice to the rest of the facility's clinicians without proper certifications or training. Veronica's role as an art therapist might be placed in jeopardy if she does not advocate for her field effectively. Eric would benefit positively from this option. Eric would remain in good standing as a counselor at the facility and his successful idea to use "art therapy" with the group would be shared in a positive light with other clinicians. The adolescents in Veronica and Eric's group would be positively affected by this option due to the continued support of an activity that they responded well to. While this continued support would be a positive outcome, if art therapy techniques are later applied incorrectly, it may bring them to harm long term and give them a misleading view of what art therapy truly is. The clinical director would benefit from this option because her clinician will remain in good standing and her thought to share this idea with the other resident clinicians would remain. The clinical director will be happy to see a successful idea become common practice with the rest of her staff. Other clinicians and staff at the facility would not be affected by this option because things would remain the same for them. The only negative outcome from this option for Eric, the clinical director, and facility staff would occur if it is later determined that they are actually practicing outside of their scope of practice. As for the other clients at the facility, they might benefit positively as long as the clinicians continue to remain within their own scope of practice when using art as a therapeutic tool.

3.2.3 A-Assistance

3.2.3.1 Assistance from Consultants

There are several questions Veronica should consider pertaining to this case. First, she must decide what is and what is not art therapy. She must consider if Eric is actually using art therapy to be able to make her decision. This is a clinical question, and she should consult her supervisor. It is likely Veronica and her supervisor will decide the coloring pages are not art therapy by themselves, but the context in which they are presented and used is important and can change whether this directive would be considered art therapy or not. Veronica should also consult her supervisor about the appropriate way to confront a coworker and clinical director. Veronica's clinical supervisor will remind her that ethical codes state an informal resolution is important if she thinks Erica and her clinical supervisor are violating ethical codes.

Veronica should also ask the other clinicians at her site what types of groups and directives they regularly run. This is important to find out if they are utilizing art therapy in a way that practices beyond their scope. The other clinicians tell Veronica that they don't run art therapy groups, but they do run creative expressions groups which involve providing art supplies and coloring pages for the youth to use as relaxation time. No processing happens during these groups. Veronica feels comfortable that these groups are not depicted as art therapy and are not violating any ethical codes. This means it may be even more important for her to discuss the use of art therapy being introduced into groups without a trained art therapist.

Veronica should also find out the official way to file an ethical complaint about a clinician. This is both a legal and risk management question due to the fact that she is worried about losing her position if she confronts her director. She should call the legal team at both of her professional organizations to acquire consultation about this process.

Lastly, Veronica should determine what the risk is to her clients if she leaves the group. This is a clinical, ethical, and risk management question. To determine this Veronica should consult with her supervisor as well as her client's primary clinicians on site. It is important for Veronica to determine this so that no harm comes to her clients if she is terminated. In discussion with her supervisor and the primary therapist of the youth, Veronica decides that Amy is the highest risk in the group, due to recent expression of suicidal ideation to her therapist. Amy has been engaging very well with the art therapy groups Veronica has done, and her therapist was hoping this trend would continue and would help Amy's suicidal ideation.

In Figure 3.3 two: assistance artwork, Veronica utilizes the metaphor of a large soup pot to imagine integrating the feedback from other professionals she will get in making this decision. Each ingredient is an important part of the final product, and she imagines how feedback from each professional will help her finalize her ethical decision as she completes this drawing.

3.2.3.2 Assistance from the Literature

It is important that Veronica not only acts in an ethical manner, but that she is acting in the best interest of her clients. Hinz (2017) states that art therapists must act in a way that promotes creativity as a basic human right and that art therapists should avoid participating in a practice that limits the creativity of their clients. Veronica must take into consideration that her actions may limit the chances of her clients participating in creative activities. At most residential facilities the clients are on a strict schedule and do not often have access to art materials outside specific groups due to safety concerns. This research supports option two, because if Veronica decides to confront Eric and her clinical director, the youth may lose access to art materials in other groups, limiting their chance to express themselves creatively.

According to Kapitan (2011), every ethical decision a practitioner makes sets into motion future choices not just for them, but also for their coworkers and the institution they work for. Veronica must take into account that her decision does not just affect her current coworkers and clients, but may affect how the residential facility and the larger company that owns them see art therapy. If she decides not to speak up, art therapy may be seen as something that can be practiced by those not licensed in art therapy, or as little more than arts and crafts that any staff member can utilize. If she advocates for art therapy being practiced only by those trained and licensed in it, then she may have a chance to educate not only her facility, but the greater organization on what art therapy is and the benefits of utilizing it for their population. This could create other jobs for art therapists in the organization, as well as other practitioners under

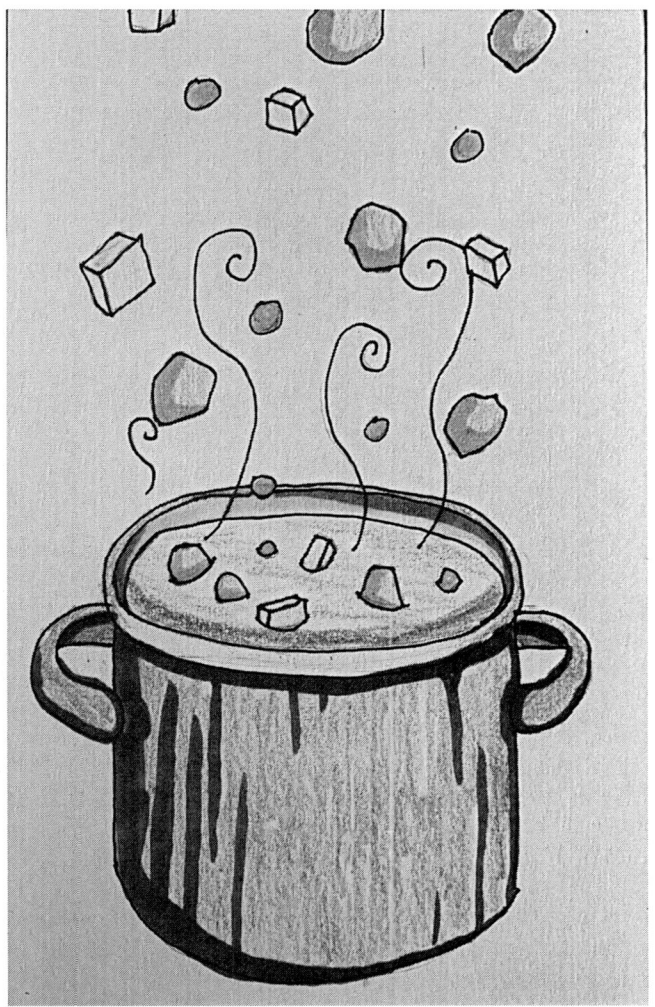

Figure 3.3 A large pot steaming and filled with ingredients illustrating the integration of the two parts of the assistance stage.

the creative arts therapy umbrella. Due to these reasons, and the potentially large impacts to her organization, this research supports option one.

According to Feen-Calligan (2012), there are several things that threatened the professional identities of art therapists including mixed messages about the status of the art therapy profession, art therapy not having billable rights, the public not understanding art therapy, credential difficulties, and employment issues. Experiences that nurtured professional identities were the relationship with mentors and faculty, pushing past their comfort zones, learning about specific populations, and finding positions that valued art therapy (Feen-Calligan, 2012). To help protect her professional identity as an art therapist and navigate her dual roles, it may be important for Veronica to utilize option one to speak out and protect her field to help protect the professional identity both for herself and other art therapists.

3.2.4 R-Responsibility/Risk

In this case, the most relevant parties that Veronica is directly responsible for would be Eric and the adolescent clients in the group that they facilitate together.

3.2.4.1 Option One

In Option One, Veronica would be fulfilling her responsibility to Eric as his coworker by directly confronting him about her valid concerns regarding his use of "art therapy". Veronica would also be fulfilling this by protecting Eric from misusing art therapy techniques and breaking ethical codes that he has agreed to uphold as a licensed counselor. However, she would not be fulfilling her responsibility to Eric by accusing him of acting outside of his scope of practice without further consulting literature and professionals within the field. Additionally, Veronica would not be fulfilling her responsibility to her mental health counseling identity where it is acceptable to utilize creativity in treatment. If Veronica was to decide to confront Eric about this option, she would need to provide Eric with evidence that shows how his idea could be seen as harmful to the art therapy field as a whole and their clients.

3.2.4.2 Option Two

In Option Two, Veronica would be fulfilling her responsibility to Eric by trusting his decision-making in order to best help their group. In addition, Veronica would be fulfilling her responsibility to the adolescents in her group by continuing to support their exploration with and use of art in their sessions. Further, this would be in alignment with her mental health counselor identity to include creativity in treatment. However, Veronica would not be fulfilling her responsibility to either Eric or the adolescent clients that she is working with by allowing Eric to continue calling his use of art in a group, "art therapy", which may lead to misconceptions about art therapy in general.

3.2.5 T-Take Action

After identifying the options available, reviewing ethical codes from appropriate organizations, considering all possible outcomes of the options, and utilizing all applicable resources, the most ethically sound choice would be Option One, confronting Eric. Even if there is a misunderstanding between Veronica and Eric, the best choice would be to address Eric for his use of what he had claimed to be "art therapy". In this option, Veronica is carrying out her responsibility as an art therapist by upholding the standards and expectations that come with practicing art therapy and having a conversation about what is or is not art therapy. This is also in alignment with her mental health counseling identity which requires her to clarify roles and seek informal resolution when ethical conflicts arise. It is up to Veronica to move forth in a professional manner when addressing her concerns with Eric so as to approach this from an educational standpoint. Both Veronica and Eric are professionals in their field(s) and as such, should understand the need, to be honest with one another about any concerns they might see. Through support from organizations and supervision alike, Veronica should be able to find a way to appropriately address this issue with Eric. By choosing this option, Veronica is simultaneously preventing further harm to clients and decreases the possibility of any potential unethical behavior by other clinicians. By choosing to confront her coworker, Veronica will be maintaining best practices as a mental health counselor and art therapist.

3.3 Summary of the Main Concerns

There are several concerns that need to be taken into account in a case that involves a dual identity and multiple ethical codes. First and foremost, it is important to have a clearly defined role for a job, and be aware of what roles other professionals fit into in the organization. It is also important to be aware of ethical codes relevant to other professions relevant to your organization. These codes may provide insight into handling conflicts and complaints.

Many settings have groups that utilize art in a non-clinical way, often involving coloring sheets or arts and crafts activities. Oftentimes art therapists work in isolation, without direct contact with other art therapists, as such, part of their role may include educating both the organization and other clinicians about art therapy. In addition to education, this could also include n having difficult conversations about the scope of practice, and advocating for the field in general.

Lastly, it is important to know who to consult both in a professional association and at the workplace when a serious ethical issue arises that may need to be reported. Oftentimes there are license-related ethical codes, organizational ethical codes, and laws that may contradict each other. In these cases, seeking input from professionals from multiple backgrounds may assist in gaining a greater understanding of where multiple identities overlap.

3.4 Tips to Avoid Pitfalls

It is easy to understand how difficult it may be to balance the multiple identities present in both the professional and personal lives of art therapists. Being difficult, it is the responsibility of the practitioner to adapt and adjust in order to best meet the standards of each of the roles they are a part of. This balance may be accomplished by continuously nurturing one's professional identity (Feen-Calligan, 2012). Seeking out activities and materials that maintain an understanding of individual identities can ensure that each role is met with care. Additionally, to avoid any misunderstandings, communication is key. By maintaining open lines of communication with others, art therapists can help maintain the boundaries needed in order for them to practice within ethical standards. A final tip would be to utilize all forms of resources, both educational and professional, in order to back up decisions and continue learning (Feen-Calligan, 2012). By seeking out help from resources that have been provided, it can reassure the therapist that their decision is supported by the fact over intuition alone. These suggestions allow for art therapists to build the confidence needed in order to wield numerous professional identities in their practice.

3.5 Suggested Further Readings

Elkis-Abuhoff, D., Gaydos, M., Rose, S., & Goldblatt, R. (2010). The impact of education and exposure on art therapist identity and perception. *Art Therapy, 27*(3), 119-126, https://doi.org/10.1080/07421656.2010.10129666

   This study of graduate students focused on how they saw their patients and how their patients saw them, and how this changed over time throughout their education. As students progress, they will need to express and manage their feelings to cope with the stressors as they develop their professional identity. The students were asked to draw how their patients saw them and how they saw their patients three times over the course of their education in supervision meetings. Results showed an increase in the importance of the supervisor relationship, self-awareness, and professional identity as students completed the program. Stress levels also increased as students got closer to graduation.

   Feen-Calligan, H. (2012). Professional identity perceptions of dual-prepared art therapy graduates. *Art Therapy, 29*(4), 150–157, https://doi.org/10.1080/07421656.2012.730027

   This qualitative study focused on the development of professional identity in art therapists who were also mental health counselors.

Professional identity is defined as the collective understanding of a profession held by its members and an individual's sense of self within their profession. One's professional identity may contribute to their commitment to the profession, career, and group affiliation. Results showed that the professional identities were most often a combination of art therapy, counseling, and teaching. Those with a dual professional identity often described a dynamic, variable, and shifting emphasis between counseling and art therapy that depended on the needs of the client.

Hinz, L. (2017). The ethics of art therapy: Promoting creativity as a force for positive change. *Art Therapy, 34*(3), 142–145, https://doi.org/1 0.1080/07421656.2017.1343073

The ethical codes for art therapists were last revised in 2013 to add creativity as a core value and include a nondiscrimination clause. This article explores creativity as being a basic human right. The author explains that creativity is promoted through the freedom of artistic expression within clients in order to facilitate a positive change. This article states that if art therapists participate in practices that knowingly or unknowingly limit participation in creativity, they are complicit in repressing a basic human right and denying clients the possibility of growth. This means that art therapists should actively work against any law that limits creative expression and work toward promoting creativity as a force for change.

Kapitan, L. (2010). Art therapists within borders: Grappling with the collective "we" of identity. *Art Therapy, 27*(3), https://doi.org/10.1080/ 07421656.2010.10129662

This study focused on a survey of 541 members of the American Art Therapy Association (AATA) to discuss the collective identity of art therapists. Collective identity is defined as an individual's cognitive, moral, and emotional connection to a larger community, practice, or institution. This article stated that collective identity is often expressed in preferences for rituals, names, symbols, relational and behavioral styles, and narratives. The supervisory relationship may be the most important factor that nurtures and shapes professional identity before art therapists enter the field and as new practitioners.

Potash, J., Mann, S., Martinez, J., Roach, A., & Wallace, N (2016). Spectrum of art therapy practice: Systematic literature review of art therapy, 1983–2014. *Art Therapy, 33*(3), 119-127, https://doi.org/10.1080/ 07421656.2016.1199242

This literature review aimed to determine where art therapists fit in the continuum of health delivery services by reviewing all publications from AATA from 1983 to 2014. The current popularity of adult coloring books and DIY art projects indicates the acceptance of the benefits of art-making. Art therapy is client-centered by promoting flexible movement within the system, and culturally competent because it can adapt to meet client expectations. It is an integrative mental health profession that can help people resolve conflicts, develop interpersonal skills, manage behavior, reduce stress, increase self-esteem and self-awareness, and facilitate the development of insight.

References

American Counseling Association. (2014). *ACA code of ethics.* https://www.counseling.org/Resources/aca-code-of-ethics.pdf

American Art Therapy Association. (2013). *Ethical principles for art therapists.* https://arttherapy.org/wp-content/uploads/2017/06/Ethical-Principles-for-Art-Therapists.pdf

Art Therapy Credentials Board, Inc. (2021). *Code of ethics, conduct, and disciplinary procedures.* https://www.atcb.org/wp-content/uploads/2020/07/ATCB-Code-of-Ethics-Conduct-DisciplinaryProcedures.pdf

Degges-White, S., & Davis, N. L. (Eds.). (2017). *Integrating the expressive arts into counseling practice.* Springer.

Feen-Calligan, H. (2012). Professional identity perceptions of dual-prepared art therapy graduates. *Art Therapy, 29*(4), 150–157, 10.1080/07421656.2012.730027

Hinz, L. (2017). The ethics of art therapy: Promoting creativity as a force for positive change. *Art Therapy, 34*(3), 142–145, 10.1080/07421656.2017.1343073

Kapitan, L. (2010). Art therapists within borders: Grappling with the collective "we" of identity. *Art Therapy, 27*(3), 10.1080/07421656.2010.10129662

Kapitan, L. (2011). "But is it Ethical?" Articulating an art therapy ethos. *Art Therapy, 28*(4), 150–151, 10.1080/07421656.2011.624930

McNiff, S. (2009). *Integrating the arts in therapy: History, theory and practice.* Springfield, IL: Charles C. Thomas.

Potash, J., Mann, S., Martinez, J., Roach, A., & Wallace, N. (2016). Spectrum of art therapy practice: Systematic literature review of art therapy, 1983–2014. *Art Therapy, 33*(3), 119–127, 10.1080/07421656.2016.1199242

Rastogi, M. (2017). *Creating a successful career in art therapy: Advising guide for psychology faculty and students.* https://teachpsych.org/resources/Documents/otrp/resources/Advising%20Guide%20for%20Art%20Therapy-edited4.docx

Rosen, C. M., & Atkins, S. S. (2014). Am I doing expressive arts therapy or creativity in counseling? *Journal of Creativity in Mental Health, 9*(2), 292–303, 10.1080/15401383.2014.906874

Van Lith, T., & Voronin, L. (2016). Practicum learnings for counseling and art therapy students: The shared and the particular. *International Journal for the Advancement of Counseling, 38*(3), 177–193. 10.1007/s10447-016-9263-x

4 The Ethics of Art Materials

Victoria Scarborough

Ethical use of art materials is an important part of art therapy. Materials, media, or mediums can take on many characteristics and each can be utilized in diverse ways. Each material's inherent qualities allow for various forms of expression and process (Orr, 2005). Mediums used in art therapy can serve each client uniquely, and the way a client may use material may transform slowly through the course of therapy or as briskly as within a single session (Case & Dalley, 1995). Art therapists and others trained to use art materials in therapeutic groups or sessions need to be aware of these inherent qualities, and have the training and knowledge of how to use each of their available materials with clients in order to use them ethically in sessions. The American Art Therapy Association (AATA)'s Ethical Principles for Art Therapists (2013) advises that therapists should not use art materials or processes that fall outside of the therapist's education, training, and experience.

Art materials can be thought of as being on a spectrum from solid materials which tend to be easier to control such as markers, colored pencils, or collage to looser or fluid materials such as paint, clay, or chalk pastels (Malchiodi, 2007). The solid materials may allow for placing thoughts and feelings onto paper in a more contained way, but can be limiting and rigid. Various fluid materials such as paints may lend themselves to more emotional expression, but can also lead to regression or decompensation in the client (Nainis, 2008). If there is no awareness or competence on the part of the facilitator, or if a therapist is practicing outside of their knowledge area with regards to materials, emotional and or physical safety could be at risk. If the chance exists for harm in a session due to negligence based on lack of proper knowledge base, then ethical issues arise as it would be in strong opposition to two of the American Art Therapy Association's core values, nonmaleficence, and beneficence. These two guiding values are among justice, creativity, fidelity and autonomy as the aspirational principles that help set the foundation for ethical work in the field. Values are in place to protect the people and communities served by art therapy (Furman, 2013; American Art Therapy Association, 2013).

DOI: 10.4324/9781003175124-4

There are varying theoretical approaches to working with clients and materials in art therapy. Therapists may select a single orientation or pull from several, based on the needs of the population in the setting. The therapeutic goals of treatment can also influence materials and approaches used with a particular client (Seiden, 2001). Seiden (2001) and Orr (2005) note how essential the correct choice of materials can be in that some materials may move the therapeutic process forward, while others may hinder it.

Materials can allow for both conscious and unconscious imagery of the client's state of being in that moment, on that day. Material choice and how the material is used may also be indicative of a client's frame of mind or affect at the moment that they are creating art, or where they are within the creative process (Case & Dalley, 1995). The Expressive Therapies Continuum (ETC) (Lusebrink, 1992) can be used as a tool to help guide material selection while also providing some containment. Hinz (2008) cautions against therapists who may not always have awareness of their own biases or blind spots toward certain materials. In these cases, it could result in those materials not being utilized or offered to clients when it may be appropriate or beneficial for the client to have them available. Limiting or not using potentially beneficial or clinically appropriate materials could be an ethical issue, especially if it impedes a client's ability to move forward in their therapeutic process. Hinz (2008) reported that she believed knowing and utilizing the ETC can help therapists avoid errors as it relates to materials.

Depending on the setting or client, some art therapists may work from more of an open studio approach and may encourage spontaneous expression. Clients may have access to nearly every material available for use in the art therapy space. Other times art therapists may work in a structured or directive-focused manner and may pre-select materials used for the individual session or group. Art therapy assessments or testing tools may also call for the use of specific materials and directives (Malchiodi, 2003). No matter the approach, the therapist needs to be working within their own scope of practice with knowledge surrounding the materials, the theoretical orientation, and any tools they are using, in order to limit risks and perform their trade in an ethical manner.

Both the American Art Therapy Association (2013) and the Art Therapy Credentials Board (2021) necessitate a safe environment for art therapy. Keeping the environment safe and secure also pertains to the materials themselves. It is imperative that art therapists not only have strong knowledge about the materials they are working with, but are aware of any potential hazards or toxicity, as well as, any safety precautions that are needed in order to keep all clients safe (Moon & Nolan, 2020). Consideration must be given to how materials are stored, and have protocols in place for safety in case of any incidence. Depending on the setting, safe storage of materials may encompass where the materials are kept, who has access to them, and at what times they are available for use in the setting. When art therapists are selecting materials they must also consider the physical space in which they will work. The therapist needs to take into account whether or not there will be access to water or a sink for clean up. The therapist should ensure that there is adequate ventilation particularly with any high fume materials (Moon & Nolan, 2020).

Maintaining a secure environment may also involve monitoring the use of materials very closely, as virtually any material could cause harm if used inappropriately. Pointedly, protocols may need to be in place for the use of sharp objects like scissors, or any object that could burn a patient such as a hot glue gun or a kiln. In certain types of mental health settings such as an acute inpatient psychiatric unit or a jail, there may be strict limitations to the types of materials that are allowed to be present in order to keep everyone safe (Moon, 2010). In having a deep under-standing of the materials, the working space, and the person or popula-tion that is utilizing them, the therapist can determine when it may be appropriate to utilize certain types of objects or media, or if it would be unsafe in a session. In medical environments, when working with im-munocompromised clients, or during national pandemics, single-use or disposable art materials may be required, and cleanliness or sterilization of shared materials is necessary (Moon, 2010; Nainis, 2008). Ethical risks would occur if infection control protocols were not enforced.

Some art therapists may feel it is important that art materials be of a certain grade or quality as it may send an unconscious message to clients if the materials are of high artistic quality versus those that are lower-quality materials. Other therapists rely more heavily on found objects, recycled materials, craft supplies, collage, or wood. The theory being that not ev-eryone can afford fine art grade materials, and that art can be made out of anything (Moon & Nolan, 2020). Further, there have historically been art therapists who have resisted certain types of materials, for example, wax crayons, that could be seen as infantilizing when offered to older clients, while others may welcome their use in various ways (Horovitz, 2018). Increasingly there has been an inclusion of technology-based materials (Orr, 2005), which can bring about their own set of ethical risks. Moon (2010) highlights how these new media are often collaborative and encourage participation, but can at times blur traditional boundaries. Therapists need to be well versed in how to maintain confidentiality and safety in these new environments (Alders et al., 2011; AATA, 2020; Moon, 2010).

Regardless of material choice, it is important that they are well orga-nized or found with ease (ATCB, 2021; American Art Therapy Association, 2013). Moon and Nolan (2020) state the ethical importance for therapists to understand the impact any material can have on clients regardless of the materials approach.

As mentioned, the potential for risk could be incurred if knowledge about the materials and their artistic properties are not present.

Therapists need to be aware when selecting any medium of potential difficulties a client may have to utilize the material whether it be from unfamiliarity with a material, sensory sensitivities, or difficulty with fine motor skills. Issues can also arise if a patient is emotionally flooded by a material or experiencing overstimulation. Art therapists' understanding of how materials are used can help them to adapt materials or the work environment to assist the client, and make it more accessible and safe (Malchiodi, 2013). Art therapists must have the ability to tailor materials as needed, to ensure media are inclusive to people of all abilities regardless of age, gender, or culture (Moon, 2010). Ethical risks could be incurred if materials are contraindicated for the setting or population of clients.

Ethical issues may also arise if there are not culturally appropriate or inclusive materials available. Moon (2010) and Hocoy (2002) reported that historically traditional art therapy materials may have aligned more heavily with Western ideals of what art should be, and may not have always been culturally appropriate or accessible to the population utilizing the therapy. Moon (2010) recommends further examination and expansion of art materials used within art therapy to meet the needs of all potential clients and advocates for an increase in publishing these practices, which would support advancement in the field. Having this type of literature available would be advantageous if ethical dilemmas arise. To remain ethically sound, therapists also need to be aware of their own culturally-based preference for materials and aesthetics, and continue to educate themselves on the multiplicity of art materials and their uses (Moon, 2010). If facilitating art therapy in another country or culture, Golub (2005) and Kalmanowitz and Lloyd (2002) advocate for not necessarily utilizing traditional art materials, but rather finding what is available locally and utilizing found objects to make art media.

Depending on the setting in which art therapy takes place, acquisition of materials may come easily with budgets set aside specifically for their purchase, or art therapists may rely more heavily on donations of materials and supplies. The types of available materials may be more limited if the therapist or agency does not have a budget for art materials. Ethical challenges could arise in relation to the procurement of materials, and in situations when materials are very limited. Bush (1997) stated when discussing art therapy programs in schools, how the procurement of monetary funds for programs and materials was often a prohibitive obstacle, and the obstacle remains in many settings today.

4.1 The Case of Jennifer

Jennifer is an art therapist working at a not-for-profit adult outpatient mental health clinic that specializes in the treatment of clients diagnosed with various types of eating disorders along with co-existing diagnoses. The clinic is located in a large urban area and services many of the diverse surrounding areas. Jennifer facilitates art therapy groups with clients who present for treatment at the intensive outpatient level of care.

Melanie is a married white female, and mother of two young children, who is in her mid-forties. She has received treatment at the outpatient clinic for the last six weeks for binge eating disorder and generalized anxiety. While Melanie is high functioning and successful in her job and as a mother, the stress and anxiety she experienced led her to attempt to cope through food. In order to focus on treatment, Melanie took leave from her job.

Over the course of treatment, Melanie has been a supportive and engaged participant in the groups she has attended while in the program. Melanie is one of the older members in the group, and has taken on a mother-type role within the group. She reports that she felt the art therapy groups have been particularly beneficial in her recovery, and felt that art-making could at times be a calming mechanism for her. She was able to use art therapy as a means for self-expression and exploration. Melanie often seemed surprised at the content that would arise for her from the art-making and through the art therapy directives.

Since there is no dedicated art therapy space within the treatment center, in running the group sessions Jennifer typically brought a set art therapy directive along with a small selection of basic art materials for the clients to choose from. Art therapy sessions took place in the dining room so that the group members could use the tables for art-making. Jennifer is conscientious of the current group's level of functioning, the designated space for the group, and the ability of clients to use materials safely when choosing the materials for the group.

As Melanie approaches discharging from the program, she expresses wanting to give some unused high-quality professional fine art supplies she has at home to the program for use in future groups at this location. While the program has a wide variety of basic art supplies at their disposal, the facility is marginally limited on materials that can be used due to not having a dedicated space or a sink nearby. Consequently, it had previously been decided at this location only basic art materials would be used.

Jennifer is unsure of how to respond to Melanie's offer because although many of the group members would probably appreciate better quality materials, this art therapy setting is not conducive to using these materials. Further, Jennifer worries how clients may respond when high-quality professional art materials are inevitably damaged, and the facility may not have the means to replace them.

4.2 Analysis of the Case

Jennifer, an art therapist, is faced with deciding whether or not it is ethical to accept the donated art materials from a client who is discharging the program. Jennifer may decide to accept the donated materials from Melanie (Option One), or to decline the donated art materials (Option Two).

4.2.1 D-Dilemma

Jennifer created artwork to aid in her decision-making process. Her first image represents her two options (see Figure 4.1). A box of watercolor paints unobstructed represents accepting the art materials, and paintbrushes, partially obstructed from view, represent declining the art materials. The codes and principles that lend weight to both accepting and declining the art materials are represented in her image through the black paint which obstructs a portion of the materials from view.

4.2.1.1 Option One: Codes and Principles supporting Option One

In Option One, Jennifer accepts the art materials from the client. The Art Therapy Credentials Board (ATCB, 2021) code 1.1.4 which states that art therapists respect the rights of their clients to make decisions, lends support for this option. The American Art Therapy Association (American Art Therapy Association, 2013) principle 1.1 also encourages art therapists to support their clients in making their own decisions, and to help clients to understand any consequences that may result based on those decisions. If Jennifer accepts Melanie's decision to provide the art materials, she should be sure Melanie understands the consequences of the decision, including the limitations of the facility and impacts on other clients.

American Art Therapy Association (2013) principle 14.6 pertains to therapists remaining attentive around termination. Jennifer would want to be sure that Melanie has a positive termination experience and that she does not regress due to the possible negative experience of her donation being declined. American Art Therapy Association (2013) principle 6.8 states that art therapists should not knowingly demean or harass anyone they interact with, which could support accepting the donation. This would be applicable if declining the materials results in the client questioning her self-worth. Refusing the donation could also be seen as demeaning to Jennifer's other group therapy clients. ATCB (2021) code 2.4.8 which references therapist considerations when presented with a gift, could also be used to support Option One if the gift or donation is deemed therapeutically appropriate for Melanie.

4.2.1.2 Option One: Codes and Principles Discouraging Option One

Since the art materials are not typical to Jennifer's scope of practice at this facility, she could be going against American Art Therapy Association

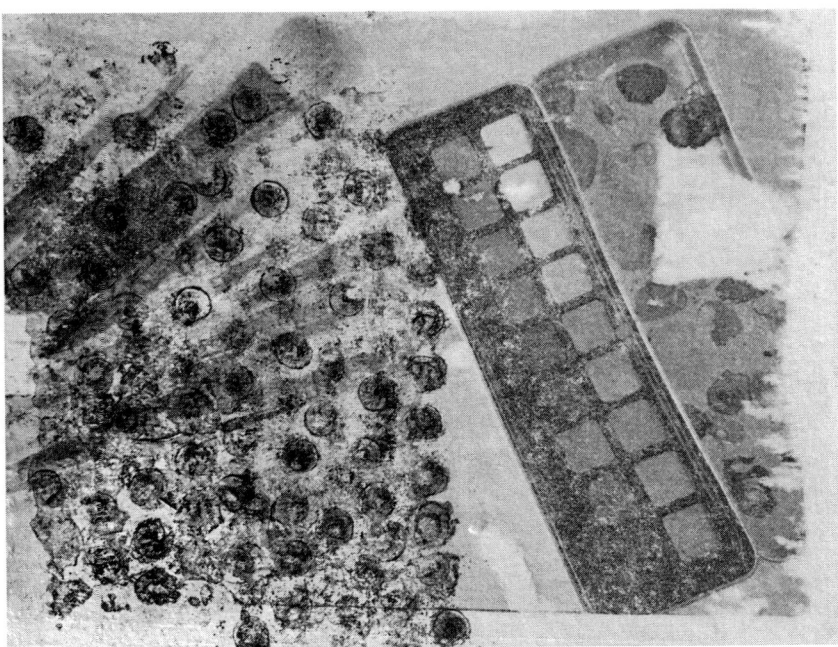

Figure 4.1 Jennifer created a visual of art materials to represent her dilemma to either accept or decline the donated art materials from her client.

(2013) principle 6.2 and ATCB (2021) code 1.1.6 pertaining to art therapist's necessity to work within their areas of experience and expertise. In addition, Jennifer may not be able to use the materials responsibly with clients given the limitations of the facility. Underscoring this is the concern that the materials may not be appropriate for the space, and may in fact pose a hazard or danger which would be in contradiction to ATCB (2021) code 1.1.14 and American Art Therapy Association (2013) principle 1.8. ATCB (2021) code 2.4.8 pertains to gift-giving and could be used to discourage accepting the fine art materials as the monetary value of the fine art supplies may be expensive.

4.2.1.3 Option Two: Codes and Principles supporting Option Two

In Option Two, Jennifer declines the art materials from the client. ATCB (2021) code 1.1.14 and American Art Therapy Association (2013) principle 1.8 outline the importance of providing a safe and functional environment for art therapy services, which includes having the knowledge and understanding surrounding the materials themselves. Since the materials Melanie would like to donate may not be appropriate for the space, Jennifer could potentially be going against what would be best for the safety of the group.

ATCB (2021) code 2.3.2 references not entering into dual relationships with current clients, former clients, close personal friends of clients, or client's families. If Jennifer accepts the fine art materials, it could possibly blur boundaries with Melanie, as she would be seen as a donor and not strictly a client. This could open up the relationship to confusion over appropriate boundaries, especially if Melanie ever returned to treatment again in the future.

Declining the art materials would also eliminate any possible perception of financial exploitation given that the materials are fine art materials and have the possibility of being expensive. ATCB code 2.4.4 and AATA principle 11.2 both explicitly state that art therapists shall not exploit clients.

4.2.1.4 Option Two: Codes and Principles Discouraging Option Two

Declining the art materials would be discouraged by ATCB (2021) code 1.1.4 and American Art Therapy Association (2013) principle 1.1 which both support the client in making her own decisions. Jennifer can advise and support in the decision-making process, and be sure Melanie understands any possible consequences, but ultimately it is Melanie's right to choose. American Art Therapy Association (2013) principle 6.8 discourages declining the art materials if the decision to turn away the donation could be viewed as demeaning to the client.

4.2.2 O-Outcomes

Those that would be affected based on the various options are Jennifer the art therapist, Melanie the discharging client who wishes to provide the art materials, the outpatient treatment facility including the facility's other staff, and other present and future clients. Jennifer created an illustration from mixed media and visually represented various types of art materials to represent the different constituents affected by the decision (see Figure 4.2). All of the materials in the image are close together, and in some cases are overlapping, representing the intertwined nature of the options and outcomes.

4.2.2.1 Option One

If Jennifer accepts the art materials the client might be positively impacted. Melanie may have positive feelings about being able to provide the art materials. She may feel that she was able to give back to the treatment center in some way, or that part of her is still there supporting

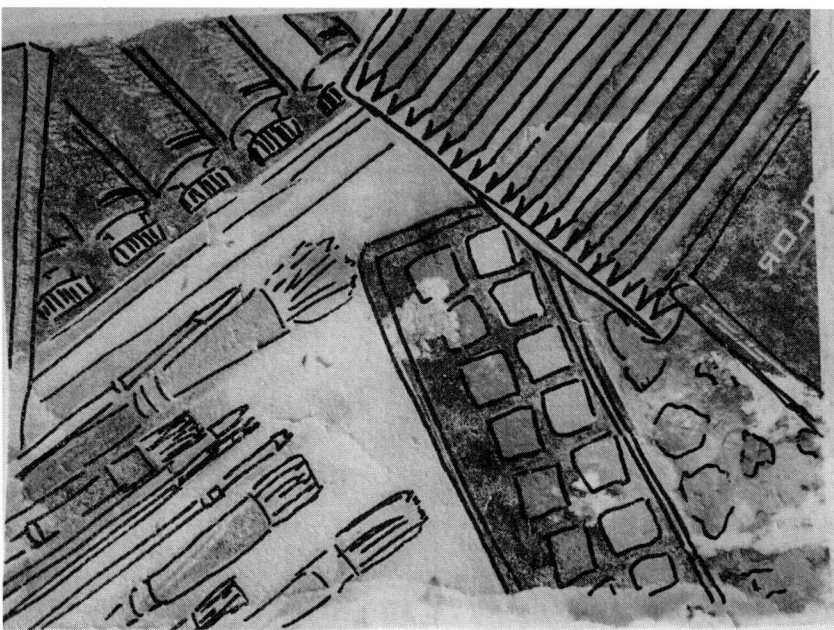

Figure 4.2 Jennifer's illustration of different types of art materials represent the various constituents affected by the options and outcomes and how they are intertwined.

her peers through the art materials. Jennifer's other current and future group members, and other staff at the facility might also benefit from receiving the materials. Specifically, they would be able to use high-quality art supplies. Other group facilitators at the treatment center may benefit from using the donated materials for other non-art therapy groups that could be enhanced from or require the use of these supplies.

However, accepting the materials could also negatively impact Jennifer and other staff, as they would need to determine how to maintain and use the materials with limited resources. Other clients could also be negatively impacted if the materials are not appropriate or safe for the other group members or the space.

4.2.2.2 Option Two

Declining the art materials may cause Melanie to regress or feel rejected. This could reframe how she feels about her time at the treatment center and she may view her experience negatively. She may also be less likely to speak highly about the program to others who could benefit from the services offered. The treatment center, other staff, and other group members could potentially miss an opportunity to add and use art materials to the facility that they may otherwise not have acquired. However, by declining the art materials, Jennifer may be maintaining a more appropriate boundary in terms of acceptable donations.

Declining the art materials allows Melanie to remain in a client role rather than a donor role. Consequently, if she were to return to treatment, issues around multiple relationships would be avoided. In addition, current clients and staff would not be perceived as engaging in favoritism or preference. If another client felt Melanie was being favored, it could negatively impact their treatment outcomes, or the overall group dynamic.

4.2.3 A-Assistance

Seeking consultation from others upholds the American Art Therapy Association (2013) principles 1.7 and 6.4 which encourage art therapists to seek support when needed, and to work with other therapists and professionals when appropriate to best support clients. Jennifer visually depicted this process of receiving assistance from consultants and literature (see Figure 4.3) with a piece containing colored pencils that represent the various sources of assistance she received both internal and external, and a butterfly representing how she took the information given, conceptualized it, and brought it forward as she advances in her decision-making process.

4.2.3.1 Assistance from Consultants

Jennifer consults with other art therapists, a supervisor, other relevant professionals, legal consultants, and her professional liability insurance organization. From her peers and supervisor, Jennifer inquired about whether or not accepting the donation would be detrimental to Melanie's termination. The peers report it could be therapeutic for Melanie to give the materials as it had come up during treatment that she tended to keep material things as well as practices that no longer serve her. Jennifer's supervisor inquired about the monetary value of the fine art supplies, and questioned if it would be too expensive for the facility to accept from a client.

Jennifer also sought legal consultation through her clinic to inquire if there are legal limits to the size and type of donations that the clinic is able to accept. The legal consultant reported that the facility was unable to accept large donations like the number of fine art materials Melanie hoped to donate. Jennifer also called her malpractice insurance to inquire if there is an increased risk in a future lawsuit if she accepts or declines the art materials on behalf of the clinic. Jennifer's insurance informed her that it would not increase her risk directly because the donation was being made to the clinic, but that the clinic may assume some risk.

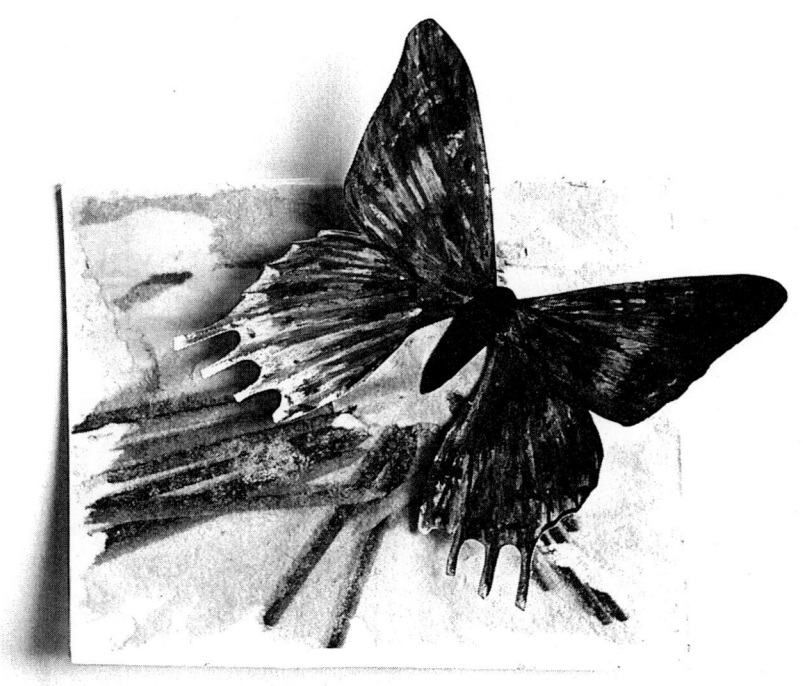

Figure 4.3 Jennifer's image represents the various sources of assistance she received and how she is able to use what she receives and conceptualize something new.

4.2.3.2 Assistance from the Literature

In thinking about the types and quality of art materials, Moon (2010) provides a historical view of art therapy materials and theory. This source reminds readers that early founders of art therapy seemed to place some importance on the use of fine art materials, and that certain materials remain somewhat dominant today in the field. Moon (2010) also looks at newer and novel mediums, and proposes viewing art therapy media, materials, and practice through a culturally competent and engaged lens. Schaverien (1992), Henley (1991), and McNiff (1998) suggest that high-quality materials can lead to higher quality expression as well as a pleasurable art-making experience, whereas poor quality materials can lead to a less invested art-making experience and consequently less commitment and pride in the art-making process. By accepting the donated fine art materials, Jennifer may be able to expand her offering of high-quality materials in the art therapy group. However, she needs to keep in mind that the facility lacks the means to store and maintain the materials. Moon (2010) and Hinz (2006) mention that some art therapists may consider whether providing too many materials at a time can lead certain populations to be less focused in their work, less appreciative of materials, and less resourceful, which discourages accepting the donation.

Given that this donation may be viewed as a gift, Furman (2013) discusses factors to consider when accepting a gift. These include but are not limited to taking into account the monetary value of the gift, being aware of any therapeutic risks or benefits associated with receiving a gift, knowing any professional or legal guidelines around gift-giving, and thinking through a client's motive for giving a gift. These guidelines lend weight toward declining the materials because of the donation's value and risk to the facility.

4.2.4 R-Responsibility/Risk

The art therapist will need to calculate potential risk to herself as well as her responsibility to each of the constituents in the case including the client, the clinic, other staff at the facility, current, and future clients. To visualize this, Jennifer created imagery of a pair of scissors within a mandala to represent wanting to cut out or reduce her level of risk, while fulfilling her responsibilities to all involved (see Figure 4.4).

4.2.4.1 Option One

If Jennifer accepts the art materials she has an increased risk of consequence or repercussions from her employer, the treatment center, if the art materials are accepted and determined to be inappropriate for the space. However, Jennifer may fulfill her responsibility and have less risk from Melanie if she accepts the art supplies, as this will likely create positive feelings regarding the donation and her termination. This may also increase Melanie's likelihood of returning to treatment in the future if she needs further support. However, if Melanie returns to treatment at this clinic in the future, there may be an increased risk since their therapeutic relationship will have been altered. Jennifer may face risk from current clients if they feel there is favoritism related to the facility accepting the donation. Clients may also enjoy and find therapeutic benefits in using the new art materials, which could fulfill Melanie's responsibilities to them.

4.2.4.2 Option Two

In Option Two, declining the art materials, Jennifer is more likely to fulfill her responsibility to her employer and less likely to create potential risks or consequences by accepting materials that are not appropriate for the setting. By declining the materials, however, Jennifer may not be

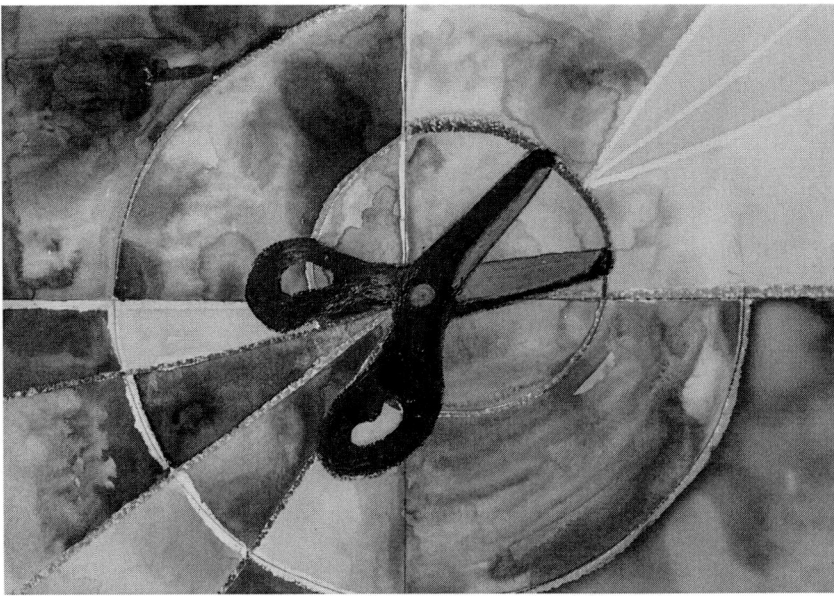

Figure 4.4 Jennifer's art represents her wanting to cut out as much risk as possible and fulfill her responsibilities to all of her constituents.

fulfilling her responsibilities to Melanie during the termination process. There may be an increased risk because of the potential negative impact on how Melanie feels about her experience in the program, and information she may share with others. Future group members would likely be unaffected and continue treatment with existing materials, which would not affect Jennifer's exposure to risk.

4.2.5 T-Take Action

After analysis of the case, Option Two, declining the art materials, is the most ethical choice. Jennifer visually represented this stage of the decision-making processing by depicting art materials that appear to be encapsulated (see Figure 4.5).

This option is supported by multiple codes and principles and allows her to maintain appropriate boundaries with Melanie. Further, the value of the fine art materials prohibits accepting the donation based on company policies. To implement this decision, Jennifer not only discussed the details of the decision with Melanie, but supported her in considering where else she could donate the unused supplies. Melanie seemed understanding of the recommendation. Jennifer documented the discussion and outcome in Melanie's therapeutic record.

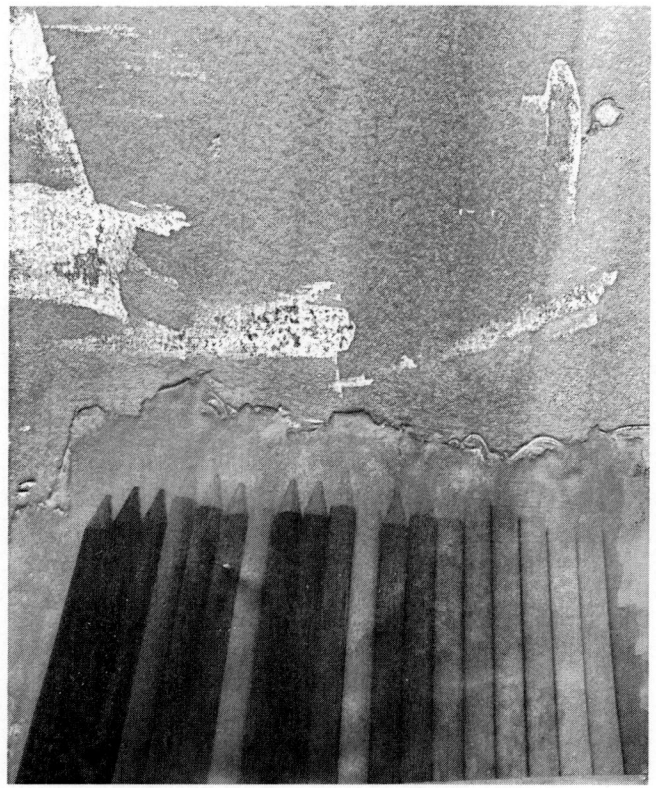

Figure 4.5 Jennifer's artwork representing her take-action step visually appears as though the colored pencils in the image are encapsulated or underneath. This represented declining the donation of fine art materials.

4.3 Summary of the Main Concerns

Art therapists need to have knowledge and understanding of the inherent qualities of the materials brought into the therapy space. When selecting materials therapists should be aware of the population they are serving, to ensure materials are congruent with the needs of the person or persons that will be utilizing them. Understanding the physical space or setting in which the therapeutic work will take place is an essential component of the material selection process to ensure materials are not only appropriate but ethical and safe.

4.4 Tips to Avoid Pitfalls

To remain ethical in the use of art materials, therapists should work with materials in which they have knowledge and training in order to remain within their scope of practice. Therapists should seek training, supervision, or consultation in areas which are outside of their personal knowledge base. Therapists can utilize tools such as the Expressive Therapies Continuum (ETC) to support their material selection process.

4.5 Suggested Further Readings

Moon, C. H. (2010). *Materials & media in art therapy: Critical understanding of diverse artistic vocabularies.* New York: Routledge. https://doi.org/10.4324/9780203858073

This book goes into detail regarding history, theory, and the use of art materials. Moon (2010) and her contributors provide examples illuminating how art materials have traditionally been used as well as some new and perhaps unconventional uses for media. The book includes a DVD or hyperlink to extra resources including colorful artwork and video clips.

Moon, B., & Nolan, E. (2020). *Ethical issues in art therapy, 4th edition.* Illinois: Charles C. Publisher, Ltd.

Ethical Issues in Art Therapy, 4th edition does a deep dive into various art therapy ethical topics including a number of mentions relating specifically to art materials and their uses within a variety of art therapy settings. To further engage the reader it includes vignettes for discussion and art directives geared toward encouraging the reader to experience these topics in different ways.

Horovitz, E. (2018). *A guide to art therapy materials, methods and applications, A practical step-by-step approach.* New York: Routledge. https://doi.org/10.4324/9781315457215

Horovitz guides readers through the benefits and contraindications of a wide number of art materials. She outlines safety implications, hazards, and precautions to consider when selecting materials that can aid the therapist in working ethically with each material. Within the text, she also provides instructions for use of art materials with consideration given to populations, human development, and art therapy assessment.

References

Alders, A., Beck, B., Allen, P., & Mosinski, B. (2011). Technology in art therapy: Ethical challenges. *Art Therapy: Journal of the American Art Therapy, 28*(4), 165–170. 10.1080/07421656.2011.622683

American Art Therapy Association. (2013). *Ethical principles for art therapists.* Author.

American Art Therapy Association. (2020). *COVID-19 resources for art therapists.* https://arttherapy.org/covid-19-resources/

Art Therapy Credentials Board. (2021). *Code of ethics, conduct, and disciplinary procedures.* https://www.atcb.org/wp-content/uploads/2020/07/ATCB-Code-of-Ethics-Conduct-DisciplinaryProcedures.pdf

Bush, J. (1997). The development of school art therapy in Dade County public schools: Implications for future change. *Art Therapy: Journal of the American Art Therapy Association, 14*(1), 9–14. 10.1080/07421656.1997.10759248

Case, C., & Dalley, T. (1995). *The handbook of art therapy.* Routledge. 10.4324/9781315779799

Furman, L. (2013). *Ethics in art therapy: Challenging topics for a complex modality.* Jessica Kingsley Publishers.

Golub, D. (2005). Social action art therapy. *Art Therapy: Journal of the American Art Therapy Association, 22*(1), 17–23. 10.1080/07421656.2005.10129467

Henley, D. R. (1991). Facilitating the development of object relations through the use of clay in art therapy. *American Journal of Art Therapy, 29*(3), 69–76. 10.12 691/education-6-7-15

Hinz, L. (2006). *Drawing from within: Using art to treat eating disorders.* Jessica Kingsley.

Hinz, L. (2008). Walking the line between passion and aaution in art therapy: Using the expressive therapies continuum to avoid therapist errors. *Art Therapy: Journal of the American Art Therapy Association, 25*(1), 38–40. 10.1 080/07421656.2008.10129352

Hocoy, D. (2002). Cross-cultural issues in art therapy. *Art Therapy: Journal of the American Art Therapy Association, 19*(4), 141–145. 10.1080/07421656.2008.1 0129352

Horovitz, E. (2018). *A guide to art therapy materials, methods and applications, a practical step-by-step approach.* Routledge. 10.4324/9781315457215

Kalmanowitz, D., & Lloyd, B. (2002). Inhabiting the uninhabitable: The use of art-making with teachers in Southwest Kosovo. *The Arts in Psychotherapy, 29*(1), 41–52. 10.1016/S0197-4556(01)00133-2

Lusebrink, V. (1992). A systems oriented approach to the expressive therapies: The expressive therapies continuum. *The Arts in Psychotherapy, 18,* 395–403. 10.1016/0197-4556(91)90051-B

Malchiodi, C. (2003). *Handbook of art therapy.* The Guilford Press.

Malchiodi, C. (2007). *The art therapy sourcebook.* McGraw-Hill.

Malchiodi, C. (2013). *Art therapy and healthcare.* The Guilford Press.

McNiff, S. (1998). *Trust the process: An artist's guide to letting go.* Shambhala.

Moon, B., & Nolan, E. (2020). *Ethical issues in art therapy, 4th edition.* Charles C. Publisher, Ltd.

Moon, C. H. (2010). *Materials & media in art therapy: Critical understanding of diverse artistic vocabularies.* Routledge. 10.4324/9780203858073

Nainis, N. (2008). Approaches to art therapy for cancer inpatients: Research and practice considerations. *Art Therapy: Journal of the American Art Therapy Association, 25*(3), 115–121. 10.1080/07421656.2008.10129597

Orr, P. (2005). Technology media: An exploration for "inherent qualities." *The Arts in Psychotherapy, 32,* 1–11. 10.1016/j.aip.2004.12.003

Schaverien, J. (1992). *The revealing image: Analytical art psychotherapy in theory and practice.* Routledge.

Seiden, D. (2001). *Mind over matter: The uses of materials in art, education, and therapy.* Magnolia Street Publishers.

5 Navigating Boundaries and Issues of Confidentiality

Mary Ellen Ruff

From the very beginning of training in the art therapy profession, the emphasis placed on maintaining boundaries in clinical work is foundational. Starting with an awareness of one's personal boundaries fosters clarity in the boundaries necessary in providing art therapy to individuals in a variety of settings. Boundaries vary in professional relationships and are impacted not only by the individual, but also by factors such as the setting, population, and culture. They can be somewhat fluid, evolving over time as the clinical relationship develops. Boundaries are also affected by technology and the limits of privacy inherent in mobile phones, the internet, and social media. Today, boundary crossings happen in many ways. At times art therapists may make a conscious decision to self-disclose either verbally or through artmaking alongside a client (Nolan, 2019). At other times, boundary crossings may occur in unexpected ways through community-based or public social interactions, with clients offering gifts to therapists, or even when clients initiate contact with therapists through social media (Zubala et al., 2021). Boundaries are also considered with regard to how the therapist navigates multiple responsibilities with clients, when and where therapy occurs, personal space, touch, and financial responsibilities (Barnett, 2017; Wilkinson et al., 2019). Art therapists must also consider that clients have a wealth of research tools at their fingertips with access to professional social media sites that highlight educational and employment history. Boundaries are dynamic and must be considered as such with careful attention to the professional roles we assume, the clinical and community settings in which we work, and the populations we serve.

The concept of dual or multiple relationships is one area that can benefit from exploration given the subtleties that can emerge within therapeutic interactions (Reamer, 2020). The focus on multiple relationships aligns with the frequency of ethical complaints that allege violations against clinicians (Boland-Prom et al., 2015; Wilkinson et al., 2019). Complaints regarding dual relationships have been the most frequently sanctioned offense across mental health disciplines (Boland-Prom et al., 2015; Wheeler & Bertram, 2015). Within the context of clinical supervision, client safety is paramount (Bernard & Goodyear, 2019). Supporting supervisee growth and clinical skill development are also significant tasks within the supervisory relationship (Dollarhide & Granello, 2016). These are important

DOI: 10.4324/9781003175124-5

considerations while focusing on maintaining boundaries within an inherently hierarchical dynamic (Cook et al., 2018). Supervisors have the responsibility of guiding newer or less experienced professionals in their clinical growth and modeling the establishment and maintenance of boundaries (Corey et al., 2020).

It is also important to reflect on the three components of ethical, legal, and risk management lenses since each can influence the action steps of a final decision. There are implications with confidentiality across each of these areas. Pope & Vasquez (2016) explore the intersectionality of these three components noting that each must be considered without one necessarily taking precedence over the others. Favoring a legal lens can lead to a stance of simply avoiding breaking the law which may not align with an ethical lens. Seeing things from a risk management perspective may lead to a more self-protective approach to art therapy which could inhibit the development of trust within the therapeutic relationship. While clinicians have an obligation to adhere to ethical codes, they must also identify the gray areas within which we practice (Pope & Vasquez, 2016). Confidentiality and its limits are defined in large part from a risk management perspective in terms of maintaining safety. Respecting this knowledge and maintaining boundaries and confidentiality are necessary from ethical, legal, and risk management perspectives.

The American Art Therapy Association *Ethical Principles for Art Therapists* (American Art Therapy Association, 2013) outlines that art therapists identify and maintain boundaries in relationships with clients through a clear definition of roles (1.3) and avoid dual relationships (1.4). In addition, art therapists are responsible to not only maintain client confidentiality but also inform clients of its limitations (2.2). Principle 15.1 addresses public information available through social media and advises that "art therapists take precautions to protect information they do not want to be available to clients," (American Art Therapy Association, 2013, p. 14). This chapter will explore the nuances of boundaries in therapeutic relationships. The case of the client turned colleague will be presented and analyzed. Images created through the discernment process are also provided to illustrate how the art therapist navigated this unexpected and unavoidable situation.

5.1 The Case of the Client Turned Colleague

Casey is an art therapist who recently transitioned from a job in an adolescent treatment center (ATC) to a position in a community mental health center (CMHC). Just before leaving the ATC, Casey worked with Sam (a teenager) and her family at the partial hospitalization level of care. Sam presented with symptoms of anxiety, depression, school refusal, and significant family conflict, particularly with her mom. Treatment consisted of group, individual, and family therapy. Over the course of treatment Casey formed a working relationship with Sam as well as both of her parents.

Sam was open in therapy and shared in an individual art therapy session that she had been smoking marijuana with friends. She indicated that she didn't believe her parents were aware of it and, despite Casey's efforts to encourage Sam to share her substance use with her parents, she refused to do so; the topic did not arise in the family art therapy sessions leaving her parents unaware of the regularity of Sam's use of marijuana. Through the course of both individual and family therapy, Sam shared her suspicions about infidelity on her father's part because of text messages she had seen on her father's phone. While Sam shared these concerns in individual sessions, her fear around her father's infidelity did not arise during the course of family therapy. Further, Sam expressed distress about her relationship with her mother, particularly regarding her mother's angry outbursts, use of alcohol, and what Sam described as her mother being "fragile." The conflict between Sam and her mother had intensified over the course of treatment and this conflict was exacerbated by Sam's father being called out of town more frequently for his job. During treatment, Sam's mother (Barbara) indicated that she was struggling to cope with current stressors and past trauma. Barbara shared that she had been hospitalized for a suicide attempt in her youth and realized in the past few months that she has continued to feel the aftereffects of a sexual assault she experienced at that time. As a result of these disclosures, Barbara was referred for her own individual therapy.

Notable in Sam's artwork was a family drawing she created expressing separation and distance between all of the family members with her mother "passed out" in a bedroom, her father, absent from the image altogether, and Sam in the woods behind her house smoking marijuana with a friend.

As treatment progressed and Casey prepared to transition to her new position in a CMHC, it was unclear whether Casey would have to transfer Sam's case to a different clinician or if she would be able to discharge Sam from the AT center's treatment program altogether. A week before her last day, Casey informed Sam and her family of her transition to a new job, and that they would have another week to work together before Casey would have to transfer Sam to another therapist to continue treatment. The family understood the situation, and Sam's mother asked Casey about her next job. Casey responded vaguely that she was moving on to a community mental health center. The family therapy session continued, and Casey felt relieved that she had not been compelled to offer more specific information about her next place of employment.

During their work together, Casey and Sam formed a close therapeutic relationship. Not only were they working individually and in family therapy, but also in daily groups including art therapy and psychoeducation. Over the course of several weeks in treatment, Sam was able to deepen her self-awareness, work with her parents on communication patterns within the family, and begin to learn and practice new coping skills for managing her emotions. She began to understand that her substance use was related to her desire to avoid intense feelings and to protect against the anxiety and discomfort within the family. Although Sam experienced some growth during treatment, challenges and frustrations remained with her parents. Similarly, Sam's parents were discouraged that her behavior had not improved more significantly. During their final individual session together, Casey and Sam exchanged artist trading cards, each reflecting upon their work together and the relationship they developed.

As Casey starts her new job at the CMHC, her supervisor informs her that she will be attending a meeting with program stakeholders involved in a community collaboration encompassing multiple agencies. Casey also learns that she will be taking over clinical supervision with a co-worker who will be at the meeting. As Casey walks into the meeting, she is both confused and surprised to see Barbara sitting at the table. Barbara looks equally surprised as neither of them was aware they would be working together, or that Casey would be providing clinical supervision for Barbara.

5.2 Analysis of the Case

The situation between Casey, Sam, Sam's family, and specifically Sam's mother, Barbara, highlights the nuances of boundaries and confidentiality that art therapists may need to navigate. Casey's awareness that she and Barbara are now colleagues as well as in a supervisory arrangement is the most pressing concern.

5.2.1 D-Dilemma

In the case of the client turned colleague, Casey is faced with the dilemma of how to transition between professional roles with Barbara while managing her own discomfort with the situation. Although she is no longer Sam's therapist, the therapeutic relationship with Sam and her family is recent and did not come to a natural conclusion due to Casey's transition to a new position. In addition, Casey is familiar with her new colleague's family history and personal challenges, which may create boundary challenges in the new supervisory dynamic. She is particularly concerned about having a multiple relationship and wonders whether she should address the potential multiple relationship with her own supervisor (which would require her to disclose confidential information about Barbara) or address it directly with Barbara (which may be difficult due to the discomfort Casey feels). To assist with processing the dilemma, Casey created artwork depicting a fork in the road (see Figure 5.1). The path appears complex to begin with and then increasingly diverges. The initial complexity of the

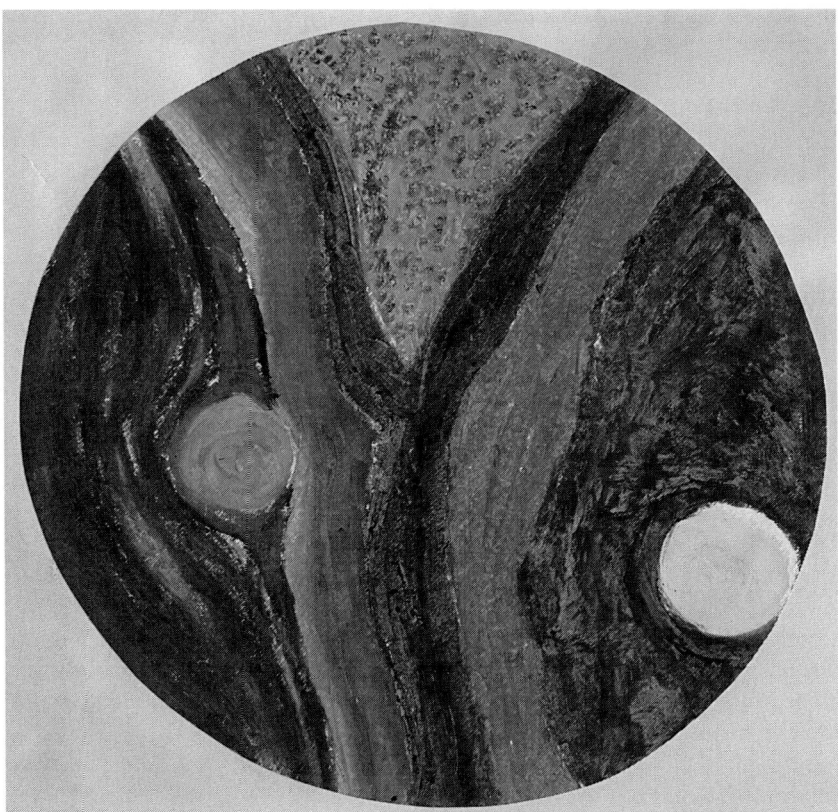

Figure 5.1 A mandala in shades of gray with a path that diverges in two directions.

path illustrates an awareness of a decision to be made with not enough information to make it immediately. This fork in the road illustrates the space that is needed to consider the options by weighing input from multiple sources in order to determine the best path forward.

The *Ethical Principles for Art Therapists* (American Art Therapy Association, 2013) and the *Code of Ethics, Conduct, and Disciplinary Procedures* (Art Therapy Credentials Board [ATCB], 2021) were consulted in identifying options for addressing this dilemma.

5.2.1.1 Option One: Principles Supporting Option One

Casey considers whether she should use supervision or consultation to address her concerns about a multiple relationship with her new colleague Barbara. AATA (2013) principle 1.7 encourages art therapists to access supervision or consultation if they experience distress or concern about issues related to clients or themselves and or if they are unclear about their own skills in managing or understanding how to proceed. Casey feels uncertain about how she should engage in a professional relationship with Barbara since she has so much personal information about the family and talking it over with her supervisor may provide support and clarity. She is also concerned that she is entering into a multiple relationship with Barbara, given her role as a former therapist, and knows that principle 1.4 indicates that art therapists "refrain from entering multiple relationships with clients," (American Art Therapy Association, 2013, p. 3). Paralleling this, ATCB (2021) code 2.3.2 also discourages art therapists from engaging in "non-therapeutic or non-professional relationships with current or former clients" (p. 7).

5.2.1.2 Option One: Codes and Principles Discouraging Option One.

As Casey weighs these options, she is aware that using supervision or consultation may not be an appropriate venue to address her concerns about entering into a multiple relationship. AATA principle 2.3 discourages her from disclosing "confidential information for the purposes of consultation or supervision without clients' explicit consent unless there is reason to believe that those clients or others are in immediate, severe danger to health or life," (American Art Therapy Association, 2013, p. 4). While Sam and her family are no longer Casey's clients, she still needs to uphold her obligations to keep protected health information confidential. ATCB (2021) code 2.1.3 also addresses the importance of maintaining client confidentiality and therefore would discourage Casey from using supervision to explore her dilemma.

5.2.1.3 Option Two: Principles Supporting Option Two

In Option Two, Casey would directly address the multiple relationship with Barbara and discuss how to navigate the evolving boundaries at work and within a supervisory construct. This is supported by principle 1.3 (American Art Therapy Association, 2013) which addresses the need to be clear about the various therapeutic roles that are possible concerning the client and therapist, and to the degree possible, prevent confusion about the boundaries and limits of the therapeutic relationship. Casey believes that if she discusses the potential role confusion with Sam's mother directly, she will minimize the ambiguity of their collegial and supervisory relationship. In addition, principle 2.3 (American Art Therapy Association, 2013) supports the need for consent in order to address client information in supervision or consultation.

5.2.1.4 Option Two: Principles Discouraging Option Two

AATA (2013) principle 8.2 and ATCB (2021) code 1.3.5 state that art therapists avoid exploiting those with whom they hold influential positions (American Art Therapy Association, 2013; ATCB, 2021). Art therapists are strongly discouraged from partaking in therapeutic relationships with either their students or supervisees. Casey is not in a current therapeutic relationship with Sam or her mother, however, she is concerned that her recent experience with the family will make it challenging to remain objective. In addition, principle 8.5 (American Art Therapy Association, 2013) addresses the disclosure of personal history on the part of supervisees, and Casey is concerned that her prior knowledge of Barbara may impact her supervision approach and the dynamic that develops between them.

5.2.2 O-Outcomes

Casey is aware that the dilemma may not only impact her, but also Sam's mother, her father and potentially Sam. In addition, there could be impacts to the new work environment and coworkers if Casey is unable to provide supervision for Barbara as per her position description. This stage of ethical decision-making creates the opportunity to sit with and reflect upon the various options that may impact a decision to move forward. To visually process the presence of options and how they impact the path ahead and the different directions that are possible, Casey created a mandala depicting several paths going in different directions (see Figure 5.2).

5.2.2.1 Option One

In using supervision to address the ethical concerns related to her new position and the responsibilities it bears, Casey is thinking not only about the impact on Barbara, but also the impact on herself, and potentially a coworker who may have to absorb the supervisory responsibilities if Casey is unable to fulfill her role in this capacity. This could lead to resentment among coworkers, particularly because the reason for a shift in responsibility might not be disclosed. By sharing her concerns in the context of supervision, she will be revealing protected health information regarding Sam's family; since she was involved in treatment as Sam's mother, Barara has a right to privacy and confidentiality. Sam's privacy is also a priority since she is the identified client and has not consented to her information being shared outside of treatment. If the art therapist were to share her concerns in supervision or consultation, she may be able to gain clarity on how to proceed professionally, but it could impact how Barbara is perceived within the workplace. If it is discovered that Casey

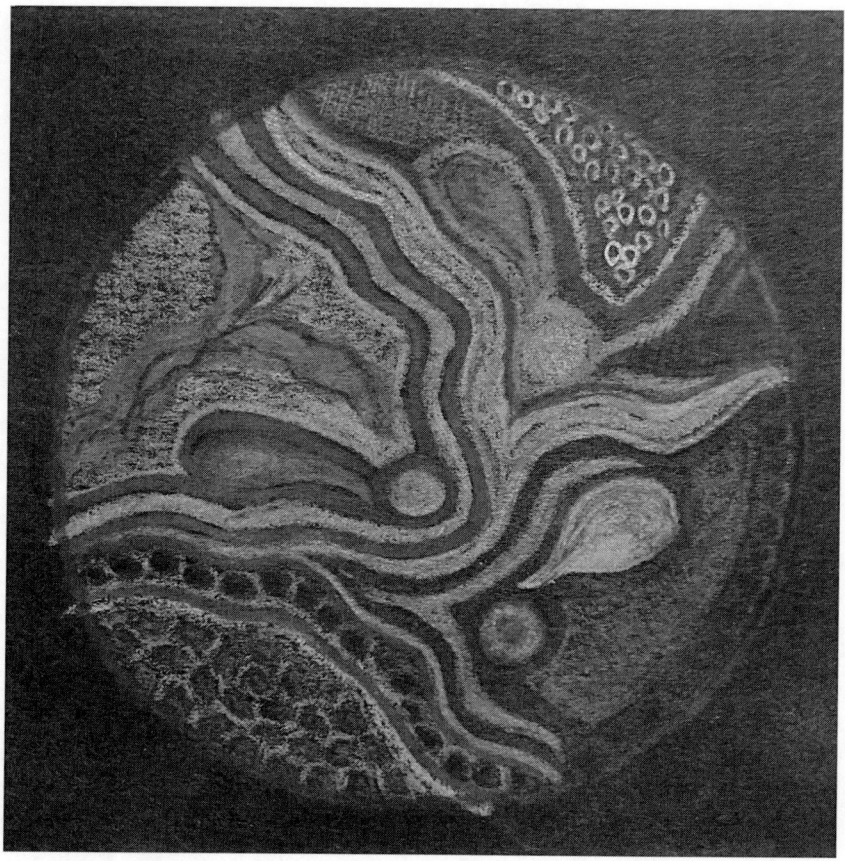

Figure 5.2 A mandala in shades of gray with several paths going in multiple different directions.

had shared protected health information without consent, it could result in an ethics complaint to the Board. Although Sam's mother may not be aware of Casey using her supervisor to discuss the situation, this doesn't condone the sharing of information without consent.

5.2.2.2 Option Two

Addressing the multiple relationship directly with Barbara may also result in consequences impacting all parties. Barbara may feel uncomfortable with her personal and professional lives commingling and this may increase her vulnerability, impact her work performance, and cause undue stress. Specifically, she may have discomfort with the knowledge that her new supervisor is intimately aware of her mental health history and current family difficulties. It may also impact the future supervisory relationship, affecting the development and maintenance of professional boundaries. By directly addressing the situation with Barbara, Casey honors her previous work with Sam and her family, and does not assume that working with Barbara will be problematic. Casey is also aware that as a new employee, she is in probationary job status, and directly addressing the multiple relationship with Barbara endorses her skill and competence in navigating ethical boundaries.

5.2.3 A-Assistance

Seeking assistance through supervision or consultation is an important support that may prove helpful when faced with an ethical dilemma. Accessing relevant and current literature, including the ethical codes, also provides assistance and should be consulted not only when faced with a dilemma, but also on a routine basis in order to stay current with advancements in art therapy. Casey visually processes this stage by depicting a bird's eye view of a person with outstretched arms, gathering information from different resources (see Figure 5.3). Cross-hatching over the whole image represents the multiple pieces of information that may be gathered from multiple sources and the intersectionality that contributes to the complexity of ethical dilemmas.

5.2.3.1 Assistance from Consultants

Consultation and supervision are both critical aspects of clinical work and should be used consistently. Having a third party, the objective viewpoint can alleviate the burden of sole responsibility for the dilemma, even if the decision and action steps remain the duty of the art therapist. Consultation can provide perspective on the dilemma and the factors that can ultimately impact the action steps taken. It is important to consider the legal, clinical, ethical, and risk management aspects of the dilemma (Behnke, 2014), and to consider whether art processes and materials may impact the chosen action. Each of these components can be considered distinctly and interdependently as part of the discernment process (Roche, 2019).

Addressing potential legal implications involves determining whether federal or state laws govern any aspect of the dilemma (e.g., Health Insurance Portability and Accountability Act [HIPAA] of 1996, Pub. L. No. 104-191). If Casey seeks supervision or consultation, is there a legal consequence in disclosing protected health information in the context of supervision or consultation without the written consent of the individual? Is there a precedent for non-routine disclosures in the context of supervision or consultation? These would be questions for an attorney or an

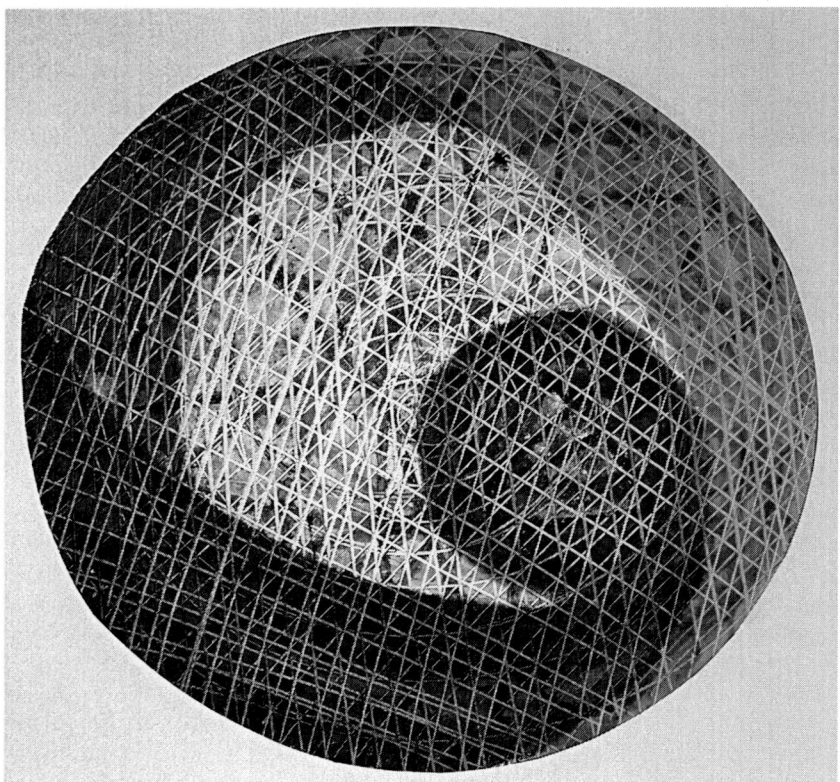

Figure 5.3 A mandala in shades of gray appearing as a bird's eye view of a head and arms reaching out for resources.

individual knowledgeable about the nuances of protected health information and the limits or legalities of disclosure. If there was a legal reason that Casey should avoid disclosing case information in the context of supervision, without consent, then she would likely choose option two and speak directly with Sam's mother.

Clinically, although Casey is no longer serving as the art therapist for Sam and her family, she must continue operating with the lens of best interest and respect, upholding the aspirational ethical values of beneficence, nonmaleficence, and fidelity. Specific questions include: Is there a negative impact on Barbara or Sam if Casey seeks supervision or consultation? Is there a clinical resource that addresses this issue of clients becoming colleagues? Talking with Sam's mother directly could negatively impact their professional relationship and Casey would not want to cause distress to the family.

The ethical lens requires a review of the applicable code and principles (i.e., AATA and ATCB). These documents provide assistance in clarifying the situations they specifically address, however, there are subtleties in many clinical situations that require some level of interpretation. Casey should look for guidance on multiple relationships with former clients, the use of supervision and consultation, consent for disclosure of protected health information, and perhaps direction regarding boundaries and self-disclosure. She must also consider the aspirational ethical values of autonomy, beneficence, nonmaleficence, justice, fidelity, and creativity (American Art Therapy Association, 2013) as a guide in considering relevant ethical questions. Specific questions would include: Will the use of supervision to discuss this dual relationship constitute a breach of trust? Is there any assurance that discussing the multiple relationship directly with Barbara will avoid undue emotional distress or will it contribute to it? While it is important to find ways to respect all of the values, tensions may also emerge when working through how each may be honored in an ethical dilemma.

Questions involving risk management are best left to experts in liability and Casey could access her professional liability insurance carrier. Questions she may ask include: can the disclosure of client information in the context of supervision be considered a breach of the standard of care or violation of client rights? If Casey chooses to talk directly with Barbara, will she be held responsible if the conversation results in emotional distress? If Barbara finds out that Casey has disclosed information related to Sam's or her own mental health issues, it could indeed cause emotional distress and potentially lead to a malpractice claim against her. However, supervision and consultation are common practices in mental health settings and are seen as being consistent with standard practice. One other question that arises relates to the point in time at which Casey is no longer bound by the consent in place at the ATC. Does she continue to be bound by the informed consent and releases of information that were in place at her former place of employment? These questions would likely be answered by the liability insurance carrier and may help Casey determine whether there is less risk in utilizing supervision without a release of information or talking directly with Sam's mother about their working relationship.

5.2.3.2 Assistance from the Literature

Consulting relevant literature is an invaluable and necessary step in the ethical decision-making process. Ethical codes evolve as professions themselves evolve, facing new and emerging factors influencing ethical decision-making (Herlihy & Dufrene, 2011). Some of the areas to consider in this dilemma include dual or multiple relationships, boundaries, and confidentiality. The roles of clinician and supervisor are also important to consider since Casey is navigating this transition. Each of these areas for consideration has aspects that are quite clear, while others are significantly nuanced. Referring to ethical codes is necessary, and further, current scholarly literature can provide research and discussion that enhances the art therapist's ability to arrive more confidently at an ethical decision.

Art therapists experience a wide range of community-based and clinical settings, some of which will adhere to a stricter medical framework while others will provide a more open and communal space of connection. Art therapists in each of these settings can experience differences in boundaries, expectations of confidentiality, and intentionality with regards to treatment planning or goal setting. Nolan (2019) discusses the range of roles and settings that have evolved in the art therapy profession, encouraging accessibility, self-awareness, connection, and growth, all of which occur across a continuum of spaces. Art therapists also have the element of the artworks that are created individually, co-created, or in a community with others. In an open studio model of art therapy (Allen, 1995), the artwork rather than the therapeutic relationship is the central focus. Understanding that boundaries may look and feel different in a context where therapeutic issues, mental or medical health, and self-disclosure are not the main catalyst for the experience.

5.2.4 R-Responsibility/Risk

Casey is concerned about the potential risks from all parties identified previously. It is important at this stage to understand the parties to whom Casey is responsible in order to assess whether each option is ethically viable. Casey has a responsibility to herself as a licensed art therapist, she has a responsibility to Sam and her family in maintaining confidentiality, and she has a responsibility to both her former and current employers since they may also bear liability depending on her actions. She is considering her responsibility to Barbara given their recent clinical history and their new supervisory relationship. She is also aware that her previous role as Sam's art therapist may become known, affecting her job duties. If Casey is unable to fulfill the supervisory component of her new job, other colleagues or her own supervisor may have to absorb that responsibility. Casey also needs to be cognizant of sharing something in the context of supervision that may change the way Barbara is perceived professionally. Casey visually processes this by depicting a figure with outstretched arms that become somewhat of a horizon line (see Figure 5.4). The arms appear to be holding up the top half of the image, indicating the weight of responsibility Casey feels in navigating this dilemma as she weighs potential courses of action.

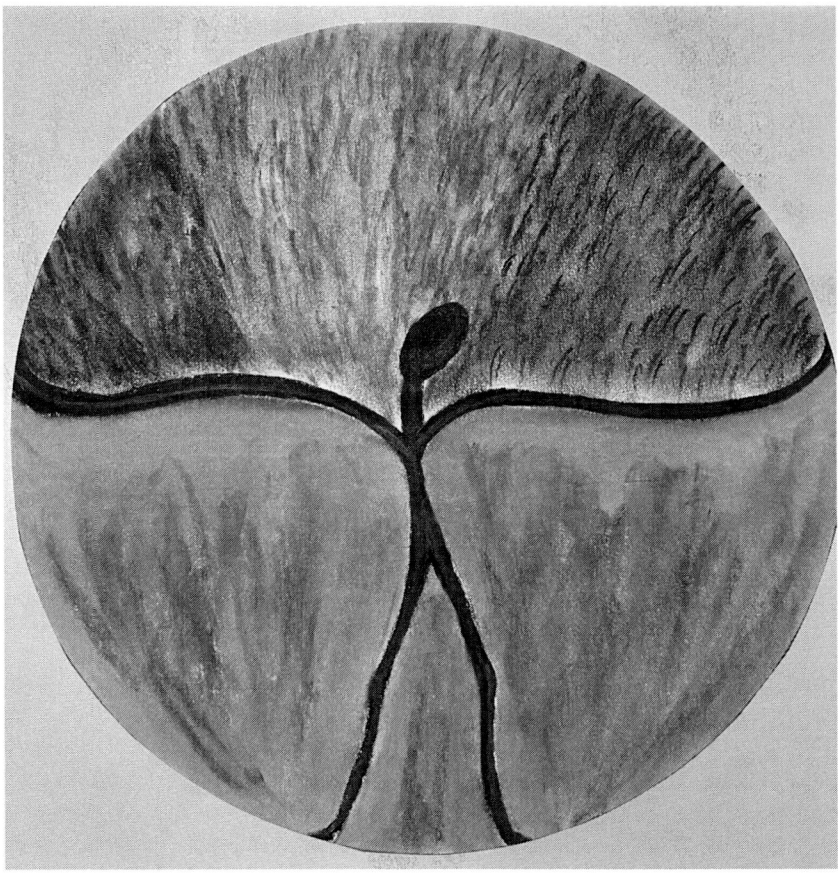

Figure 5.4 A mandala in shades of gray displaying a figure with outstretched arms as if holding up the top half of the mandala.

5.2.4.1 Option One

In this option, Casey is at risk of violating client confidentiality if she shares her concerns about Barbara with her supervisor. There is a risk of an ethics complaint against Casey which could be filed by Barbara as well as her new employer if it was felt she was violating confidentiality. In addition, Barbara may also allege a HIPAA violation which becomes a legal matter and could result in a hefty fine. The ATC is potentially liable since Casey was employed there at the time she was providing art therapy services to Sam and her family. A legal matter or ethics violation could also impact her current employer since her art therapy license could be affected, making her ineligible to hold her new position.

5.2.4.2 Option Two

The potential responsibilities and risks in this option may be different. She is still bound by HIPAA and she has an ethical duty to maintain client confidentiality. If Casey talks directly to Barbara, she is not violating confidentiality but is concerned she will cause undue stress on the new professional relationship. It could also create emotional distress for Barbara with the awareness of her own mental health history now known within her professional world. Casey has a responsibility to herself and is trying to determine her own boundaries within the situation as well. She is unsure she will feel comfortable providing supervision to Barbara given the nature and amount of information she feels she will need to compartmentalize in order to fulfill her supervisory role and responsibilities. Casey wonders whether initiating contact with a former client is an ethical violation that could result in an ethics complaint from Barbara. There is also a lingering concern that Sam's parents were not entirely satisfied with Casey's family art therapy services and wonders about potential repercussions, whether ethical or legal.

5.2.5 T-Take Action

After working through the first four steps of the ethical decision-making model, it appears as though Option 2 is the most ethical choice. Casey visually processes this by depicting a path forward with stepping stones between the foreground and horizon line, signifying the options for movement in either direction (see Figure 5.5). The sky filled with swirls also connotes the dynamic process of arriving at a place of action.

Option 2 honors several of the aspirational ethical principles including autonomy, beneficence, fidelity, and justice. It also may honor nonmaleficence although without knowing how Barbara may react, it is difficult to predict. Honoring creativity may emerge if Casey is able to work with Barbara in identifying and implementing a plan for their professional relationship. Option 2 may have a favorable impact on the supervisory relationship as a result of Casey's trust with Barbara. This could also result in a positive effect within the workplace and models respect and concern for the individual. Current literature highlights the importance of modeling ethical behavior within the supervisory relationship (Bernard & Goodyear, 2019; Corey et al., 2020). By choosing Option 2, Casey is respecting Barbara and their shared clinical experience as clients and therapists, as well as their new relationship as supervisor and supervisee, and colleagues.

5.3 Summary of the Main Concerns

Honoring the confidentiality of clients while also maintaining professional boundaries in a supervisory and professional relationship can create tension

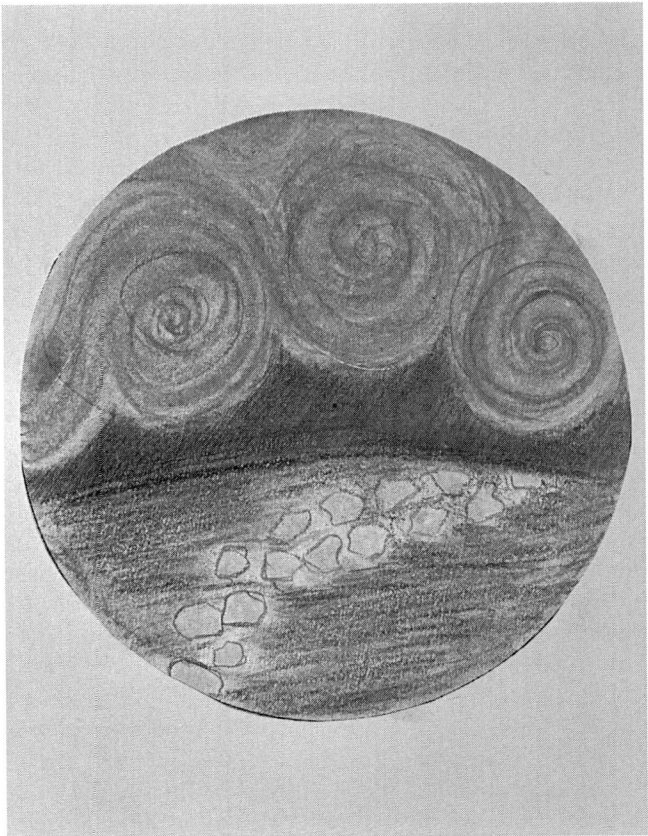

Figure 5.5 A mandala in shades of gray displaying a landscape with a clear stone
     path stretching from the foreground edge to the horizon line.

that needs to be carefully considered. The options of using supervision or
consultation and talking directly with the client/supervisee explored the
potentialities of each. Maintaining client confidentiality is paramount, and a
case such as the one described here, of unavoidable multiple relationships,
requires careful attention to boundaries. Communities can become smaller
and smaller over time and art therapy is no exception. Awareness of both
personal and professional boundaries helps art therapists prepare for the
dynamics of client relationships and the ethical challenges they may face
within them.

   As art therapists, we have the ability to engage in supervision and
consultation throughout our practice. Supervision is an essential component of credentialing and licensure and art therapists who work toward
this goal know the benefit and importance of the supervisory relationship.

This relationship also relies on the consent of clients who may be discussed in the context of supervision or consultation. The confidentiality and boundaries that are upheld in supervision enable a client to fully engage in the therapeutic process and make use of the clinical relationship. While boundaries and confidentiality seem clear and straightforward, there are myriad shades between clear and opaque, and ethical dilemmas related to boundaries and confidentiality will emerge in unexpected ways. Awareness of the available resources, the ethical codes, the expertise of supervisors, and having the willingness to actively engage with the dilemma is what strengthens art therapists individually and collectively.

5.4 Tips for Avoiding Pitfalls

Following the ethical codes, consulting and seeking supervision, and researching current literature are all important components of practicing as a professional art therapist. Ethical dilemmas are unavoidable and will often emerge from unlikely places. Thinking through the ethical, legal, clinical, risk management, and creative lenses encourages a broader, more dimensional perspective in navigating the nuances of boundaries and confidentiality that are part of clinical work. Using an ethical decision-making model can help art therapists systematically address the presenting dilemma through a series of cognitive and creative steps. Reviewing the AATA Code of Ethics (2013) and the ATCB Code of Ethics, Conduct, and Disciplinary Procedures (2021) is the important starting point for any art therapist faced with an ethical dilemma. Since many ethical dilemmas are individually and collectively interpreted, it is also important to use supervision or consultation as well as current scholarly literature for insight and additional information that may assist in making a final decision.

At many points throughout the experience with clients, art therapists may serve in many roles as they create space for the client, provide materials, assist with technical art-making processes, and in clinical settings, contribute to treatment planning and goal-setting (Moon & Nolan, 2020). Art therapists can prepare for these potential diffuse boundaries by clarifying their specific roles or roles within a setting, understanding the mission and values of the setting, and talking with their supervisor, coworkers, and clients about role expectations and limitations.

Interactions with art products are another important boundary consideration for art therapists. Malchiodi (1995) asked the important question about ownership of art created in the context of art therapy. While there are still differing viewpoints on this subject, the digital age has both simplified and complicated the storage and use of art products. Principle 4.1.a (American Art Therapy Association, 2013) ensures that clients are made aware of the inclusion of any digital or photographic copies of their artwork in their health record. Moon and Nolan (2020) discuss the spectrum of thought within the profession ranging from a strong belief in the client's ownership of the art to the important consideration of client artwork within the context of therapy records. Art therapists must be clear about the role of client artwork within the therapeutic relationship and environment as well as their limitations with regard to the storage, maintenance, reproduction, or destruction of such work.

Principle 15.0 (American Art Therapy Association, 2013) addresses the use of technology including digital and social media. Art therapists must be cognizant of the appropriateness of using technology-assisted treatment with their clients, engaging in a thorough informed consent process, and ensuring that clients are aware of the limits to privacy and confidentiality inherent in technology use (American Art Therapy Association, 2013; Choe & Carlton, 2019). Limitations noted include privacy with regards to space as well as potential disruptions in technology service or connectivity (Levy et al., 2018). More than ever, technology has increased the accessibility of art therapy, expanding the reach not only geographically, but also with the integration of technological advancements (Zubala et al., 2021). The use of technology must be thoughtful and with the best interest of the client at the forefront (Principle 15.3, American Art Therapy Association, 2013).

Ethical dilemmas involving boundaries and confidentiality occur frequently and in ways that may be unanticipated and unavoidable. From the informed consent process to the choice of materials, techniques, and space, art therapists are constantly navigating boundaries. Art therapists must be open to the available resources including ethical codes, supervision, consultation, using ethical decision-making models, and art-making to assist with carefully proceeding.

5.5 Suggested Further Readings

Green, A. R. (2012). Ethical considerations in art therapy. *Canadian Art Therapy Association Journal*, *25*(2), 16–21. https://doi.org/10.1080/08322473.2012.11415567

In this article, Green discusses the nuances of ethics specific to art therapy as opposed to other mental health professions and the overlap of ethical principles. Art therapy involves not only the client and art therapist but also the artworks created in the context of art therapy. Green notes the spectrum of voices related to the interpretation of client artwork, whether these works should be exhibited, how records including artwork are kept, and who owns the art. These important ethical questions involving client confidentiality and boundaries are thoroughly discussed.

Nolan, E. (2019). Opening art therapy thresholds: Mechanisms that influence change in the community art therapy studio. *Art Therapy*, *36*(2), 77–85. https://doi.org/10.1080/07421656.2019.1618177

This article highlights the importance of community-based art therapy studios and how the experience of participating in this setting may look and feel different than what is considered more clinical art therapy settings or even open art studios. She goes on to highlight the importance of self-awareness as art therapists in community-based art settings or art therapy studios may be creating art with clients, unintentionally self-disclosing and impacting individual boundaries.

Zubala, A., Kennell, N., & Hackett, S. (2021). Art therapy in the digital world: An integrative review of current practice and future directions. *Frontiers in Psychology, 12,* 1091. http://doi.org/10.3389/fpsyg.2021.600070

This article provides a comprehensive and updated review of literature in the art therapy profession focused on the use of digital media, particularly regarding informed consent and awareness of risks to confidentiality and boundaries. Key aspects of this article include an exploration of the range of tools and techniques that art therapists are using involving technology and the risks and benefits of these tools. One important area to explore further is the experience of clients who participate in digital or technology-based art therapy and the assumptions that are often made about access and proficiency.

References

Allen, P. B. (1995). Coyote comes in from the cold: The evolution of the open studio concept. *Art Therapy: Journal of the American Art Therapy Association, 12,* 161–166. 10.1080/07421656.1995.10759153

American Art Therapy Association. (2013). *Ethical principles for art therapists.* https://arttherapy.org/wp-content/uploads/2017/06/Ethical-Principles-for-Art-Therapists.pdf

Art Therapy Credentials Board. (2021). *Code of ethics, conduct, and disciplinary procedures.* https://www.atcb.org/resource/pdf/ATCB-Code-of-Ethics-Conduct-DisciplinaryProcedures.pdf

Barnett, J. E. (2017). *An introduction to boundaries and multiple relationships for psychotherapists: Issues, challenges, and recommendations.* In O. Zur (Ed.), *Multiple relationships in psychotherapy and counseling: Unavoidable, common, and mandatory dual relations in therapy* (pp. 17–29). Routledge/Taylor & Francis Group.

Behnke, S. (2014). What kind of issue is it? A "four-bin" approach to ethics consultation is helpful in practice settings. *Monitor on Psychology, 45,* 62–63.

Bernard, J. M., & Goodyear, R. K. (2019). *Fundamentals of clinical supervision* (6th ed.). Pearson Education.

Boland-Prom, K., Johnson, J., & Gunaganti, G. (2015). Sanctioning patterns of social work licensing boards, 2000–2009. *Journal of Human Behavior in the Social Environment, 25*(2), 126–136. 10.1080/10911359.2014.947464

Choe, N. S., & Carlton, N. R. (2019). Behind the screens: Informed consent and digital literacy in art therapy. *Art Therapy, 36*(1), 15–21. 10.1080/07421656.2019.1565060

Cook, R. M., McKibben, W. B., & Wind, S. A. (2018). Supervisee perception of power in clinical supervision: The power dynamics in supervision scale. *Training and Education in Professional Psychology, 12*(3), 188–195. 10.1037/tep0000201

Corey, G., Haynes, R. H., Moulton, P., & Muratori, M. (2020). *Clinical supervision in the helping professions: A practical guide*. John Wiley & Sons.

Dollarhide, C. T., & Granello, D. H. (2016). Humanistic perspectives on counselor education and supervision. In M. B. Scholl, S. A. McGowan, & J. T. Hansen (Eds.), *Humanistic Perspectives on Contemporary Counseling Issues* (pp. 277–306). Routledge.

Herlihy, B., & Dufrene, R. L. (2011). Current and emerging ethical is-sues in counseling: A Delphi study of expert opinions. *Counseling and Values, 56*, 10–24. 10.1002/j.2161-007X.2011.tb01028.x

Health Insurance Portability and Accountability Act. Pub. L. No. 104-191, § 264, 110 Stat.1936

Levy, C. E., Spooner, H., Lee, J. B., Sonke, J., Myers, K., & Snow, E. (2018). Telehealth-based creative arts therapy: Transforming mental health and re-habilitation care for rural veterans. *The Arts in Psychotherapy, 57*, 20–26. 10.1016/j.aip.2017.08.010

Malchiodi, C. A. (1995). Who owns the art? *Art Therapy: Journal of the American Art Therapy Association, 12*(1), 2–3. 10.1080/07421656.1993.10759011

Moon, B. L., & Nolan, E. G. (2020). *Ethical issues in art therapy*. Charles C. Thomas.

Nolan, E. (2019). Opening art therapy thresholds: Mechanisms that influence change in the community art therapy studio. *Art Therapy, 36*(2), 77–85. 10.1080/07421656.2019.1618177

Pope, K. S., & Vasquez, M. J. T. (2016). *Ethics in psychotherapy and counseling: A practical guide* (4th ed.). Hoboken, NJ: John Wiley & Sons, Inc.

Reamer, F. G. (2020). *Boundary issues and dual relationships in the human services*. Columbia University Press.

Roche, A. I. (2019). Testing for testamentary capacity in the older adult: A model of ethical considerations for the clinical neuropsychologist. *Frontiers in Psychology, 10*, 1905. 10.3389/fpsyg.2019.01905

Wheeler, A. M., & Bertram, B. (2015). *The counselor and the law: A guide to legal and ethical practice* (7th ed.). American Counseling Association.

Wilkinson, T., Smith, D., & Wimberly, R. (2019). Trends in ethical complaints leading to professional counseling licensing boards disciplinary actions. *Journal of Counseling & Development, 97*(1), 98–104. 10.1002/jcad.12239

Zubala, A., Kennell, N., & Hackett, S. (2021). Art therapy in the digital world: An integrative review of current practice and future directions. *Frontiers in Psychology, 12*, 1091. 10.3389/fpsyg.2021.600070

6 Art-based Assessment

Michele Marotta and Monica Wright

Art-based assessments are an important aspect of art therapy treatment and may be used for better understanding a client, gathering information to formulate a treatment plan. The assessment process allows the therapist to observe a number of client factors, including strengths, weaknesses, reaction to certain media, how the task is completed, and overall suitability for the continuation of art therapy (Kaplan, 2003). There are ongoing assessments and tools being developed and used in the practice of art therapy. With the rise in art assessments, it is important that these measures are conducted ethically. For example, assessments should not be used to construct an absolute diagnosis. It is also important that assessments demonstrate strong psychometric properties. Popular directives with strong reliability and validity include "House Tree Person (Buck, 1948; Kato & Suzuk, 2016)" and "Draw a Person (Naglieri et al., 1991; Naglieri 2004)." However, directives that are less prescriptive can still be beneficial. Regardless of the assessment used, a key component of the assessment is that the art is created in front of the therapist and in conjunction with a thorough explanation. This ensures that the therapist does not impose their own narrative onto the artwork.

Several ethical concerns are related to how assessments are chosen and the clients' overall comfort level with the materials or assessment itself. A factor to be considered is the client's physical and mental wellbeing. If the client is medicated or their mood is substantially impacted, they may feel less compelled to be creative or simply not have the physical capacity to do so (McNiff, 2012). Another important ethical factor to consider is the cultural and developmental implications of an assessment for the client. When selecting an assessment measure, it is important to select an assessment that is culturally appropriate for the client in much the same way that art therapists would give a client materials that are age-appropriate. For example, when selecting a measure, it is important to consider if the assessment is appropriate for the client's developmental stage. The Bird's Nest Assessment (BND; Kaiser, 1996, 2016) and its variations, including the Bird's Nest Drawing (Kaplan, 2003), measures attachment security through the task of drawing a bird's nest, is an

DOI: 10.4324/9781003175124-6

appropriate assessment tool for children and adolescents to measure attachment. However, the validity may decrease if used to assess attachment in adults (Kaplan, 2003). This assessment provides imagery for understanding the cognitive, emotional, and behavioral considerations of early childhood experiences. An advantage of The Birds Nest is that it comes off less invasive and less intense to a child than asking them to simply draw their family (Harmon-Walker & Kaiser, 2015; Kaiser, 2016). The assessment provides insight into the structure of the nest itself, the presence of nurturing figures or lack thereof. The tool has been proven reliable especially when used with the client's explanation of what they had created. The BND was created to signify images related to safety, space, and attachment. Along with the BND, a coding system was developed used to measure validity over a span of 20 years (Kaiser & Deaver, 2009). Specifically, the validity research focused on how the rating scales connected adolescent measurements with adult attachment constructs (Harmon-Walker & Kaiser, 2015). It is important to understand the research and use assessment methods with reliability and validity to know that an assessment method is measuring what it is intended to, consistently and competently.

While the creative openness of art-making is what makes art therapy therapeutic, it also leaves room for ethical dilemmas in assessment. Art is highly individual for each client and as such, ethical assessment must involve art created in therapy, alongside the therapist, in conjunction with client input. Not only is this important for ethical reasons, but the process gives insight into client experiences, mental and emotional while completing the assessment (McNiff, 2012). Much can be explored and learned simply through the creation of art with a client and the assessments formalize this process. When conducted ethically, art-based assessment can increase understanding of the client's current or past mental state.

6.1 The Case of Therapist Brown's Assessment Quandary

Brown is an art therapist who has limited experience in assessments and works in a group practice. His current client, Lydia, has expressed interest in art-making as a leisure activity and as such Therapist Brown decided it would be a good idea to start incorporating more art-making assessments with her. After looking up some assessments to use, he decided on using the Bird's Nest Drawing. Therapist Brown compared Lydia's drawing to what he read about interpreting the Birds Nest Drawing, without seeking explanations from her about the content of what she created. Brown felt the session was a great success and raved about his good experience to his clinical director Jane, who is a non-art therapist. After hearing this, Jane instructs Brown to train the rest of the clinical team in the Bird's Nest Drawing assessment. Brown recognizes that the team consists of both art therapists and non-art therapists. He is feeling conflicted and unsure of how to handle this.

6.2 Analysis of the Case

Art therapist Brown is faced with deciding if he should refuse to conduct the training on the BND, or proceed with a disclaimer that only trained art therapists can use it. Each option must consider various principles and codes. Specifically, there are a number of principles in the American Art Therapy Association (AATA, 2013) and Art Therapy Credentials Board (ATCB, 2021) that are relevant for this case. This includes principles related to ethical art therapy practice including the best interests of the client. Assessment, confidentiality, and competency-related principles are also relevant.

6.2.1 D-Dilemma

To aid in the process of understanding the dilemma, Brown used an art directive placing codes onto a set of continuum lines as shown in Figure 6.1. On one side is option one, where Brown refuses to conduct the BND training. On the other side of the continuum is option two where Brown proceeds with the training but provides clarification on training/experience needed to conduct the assessment.

6.2.1.1 Option One: Principles Supporting Option One

Option one, where Brown refuses to conduct the BND training, is supported by several principles. First and foremost, 1.0 says that art therapists have a responsibility to their clients to ensure services are being used properly and this includes ensuring proper assessment methods are used (American Art Therapy Association, 2013). In addition, art therapists have a duty to uphold ethical standards related to competence, 1.2.3 says that art therapists shall assess, treat, or advise only in areas of which their training gives them competence (ATCB, 2021). Likewise, 3.1, and 3.2 address how assessment measures may only be used with the proper application, competence, and not misinterpret results which may be put at risk when conducting the training as requested (American Art Therapy Association, 2013).

6.2.1.2 Option One: Codes and Principles Discouraging Option One

Although there are many principles that support option one, there are also several that discourage Brown's refusal to conduct the training. If Brown refuses the training he is disregarding that some participants are art therapists and they would be missing out on furthering their education and scope of practice. Principle 10.5 states that art therapists value participation in activities that contribute to bettering a community, and

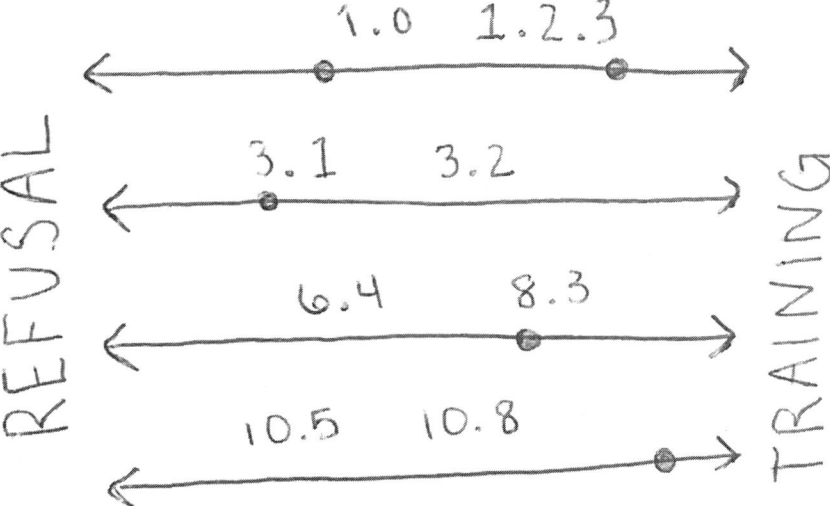

Figure 6.1 Continuum lines as a visual representation of the dilemma step.

implementing the training could do so (American Art Therapy Association, 2013). Similarly, Principle 10.8 states that art therapists are expected to take the necessary steps to prevent any misuse of art therapy findings in any agency where they are employed (American Art Therapy Association, 2013). If Brown refuses the training, then he is missing out on that opportunity to provide clarification on who can use the BND. Lastly, Principle 8.3 says that when training one must take steps to ensure employees do not perform or present themselves as competent in certain services beyond the scope of their level of experience or education (American Art Therapy Association, 2013). By the refusal of the training, Brown will be unable to ensure that this is not taking place.

6.2.1.3 Option Two: Principles Supporting Option Two

If Brown were to proceed with the training, but provide clarification on training/experience needed to conduct the assessment, there are a number of principles supporting this decision. Principle 10.5 states that it is an art therapist's duty to contribute to activities that will better a community or society (American Art Therapy Association, 2013), and by performing the training Brown will be doing so. Principles 10.8 and 8.3 all speak to how it is an art therapist's role to ensure that there is no misuse of assessment or other services beyond a scope of expertise or competence (American Art Therapy Association, 2013). Likewise, Principle 6.4 explains that art therapists must cooperate with other professionals in order to serve their clients effectively (American Art Therapy Association, 2013). In this scenario, Brown is conducting the training with the appropriate disclaimers to ensure that clients are not improperly assessed. If Brown were to provide the training, he would be able to further the current art therapist's education and training, and also ensure that the other non-art therapist's counselors are aware of the limits of their competence needed to conduct the BND.

6.2.1.4 Option Two: Principles Discouraging Option Two

`Various principles discourage proceeding with the training. Principle 1.0, regarding the responsibility to clients, ensures that services are being used properly, and if Brown trains the employees there is a chance services will be misused (American Art Therapy Association, 2013). Similarly, ATCB (2021) code 1.2.3 addresses the importance of competence in assessment, treatment, or advice. Likewise, Principle 3.1, and 3.2 address how assessment measures may only be used with the proper competence which complicates matters since Brown is a novice with the BND (American Art Therapy Association, 2013).

6.2.2 O-Outcomes

In this case, the relevant parties are the art therapist Brown, the Clinical Director Jane, the client Lydia, professional colleagues at the practice, and future clients of the practice. All of these parties are impacted regardless of which option is taken. This stage asks art therapists to think about the potential outcomes of each option by considering how the relevant parties are affected. Brown engaged in art-making to process the outcomes, and created a representation of Libra scales, weighing option one and option two (see Figure 6.2). In this image is a feather on one side of the scales, representing the consequences of option two. On the other side of the libra, scale is a pile of pebbles, symbolizing the weight of the consequences in option one. It is important to weigh the foreseeable consequences, both desirable and undesirable, through a utilitarian lens to all parties involved in the scenario.

6.2.2.1 Option One

If Brown refuses to conduct the training, it could potentially impact him, his current and future clients, and the other art therapists in the practice. Lydia and future clients would avoid the potential harm that would occur with untrained art therapists or clinicians who are not art therapists using art therapy assessments. Brown, however, may face undesirable consequences from his Clinical Director Jane who may be upset at Brown's refusal to conduct the training. This could potentially harm Brown's reputation and put his job at risk. Furthermore, other art therapists in the

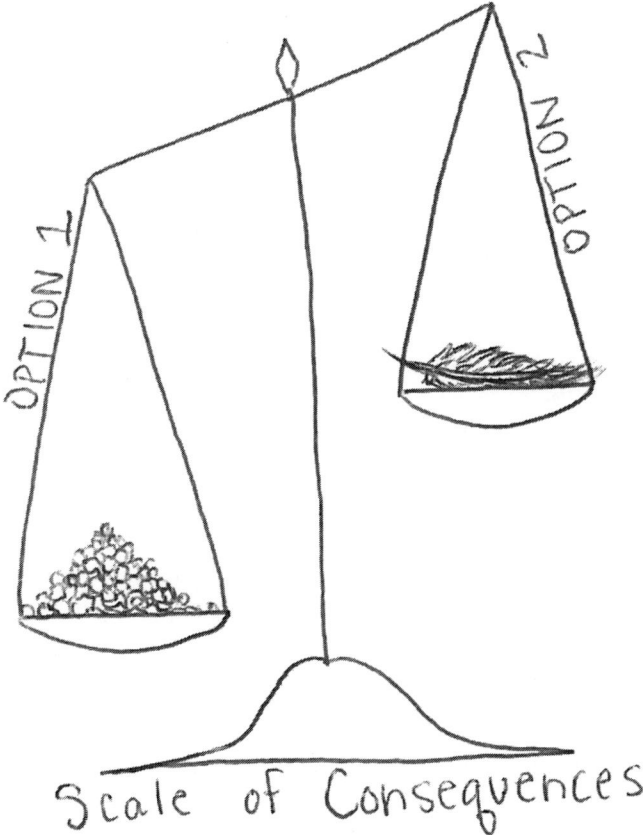

Figure 6.2 Outcomes represented by a libra scale.

practice may be negatively impacted because they will not receive training to further their competence in art therapy techniques.

6.2.2.2 Option Two

The option to perform the training but provide a disclaimer about the credentials and experience needed to competently use this assessment would also impact all parties involved. The art therapists in the practice would greatly benefit from the further training and Jane would be appeased. Lydia and future clients may also benefit as clinicians would have an expanded repertoire. However, Brown would be implicated should the assessments be used improperly and he may face negative repercussions. He may be able to avoid these negative consequences if he effectively stresses the importance of competence about who can and cannot use these assessments.

6.2.3 A-Assistance

Consultation can be a valuable tool for art therapists to utilize when faced with complicated decisions. Some resources include consulting colleagues, supervisors, professional boards, and ethical codes to gain more information and answers regarding the case. Other forms of resources include literature and research related to the case. To aid Brown in the process of taking action on a decision, he utilized an art directive representing the different assisting parts from consultants and literature and how they contribute to the decision-making process. Depicted is a funnel where questions are filtered through assistance from consultants and literature in order to aid in the decision process (see Figure 6.3).

6.2.3.1 Assistance from Consultants

There are several questions Brown may ask to gain insight into the ethical decision. A risk management question that Brown may have is "are there professional risks to conducting an assessment training knowing some participants don't have the required credentials to utilize the assessment in practice?" In consulting a supervisor, colleague, or attorney, the answer to this question is likely yes, that there are professional risks teaching a technique that may lead to assessment misuse. This answer lends support to Brown refusing to conduct the training.

Another clinical question Brown could have is "could conducting the assessment training have a negative impact on clients?" A clinical question like this could be best answered by a supervisor. The most foreseeable answer is no, Brown offering the training would not have a negative impact on his clients. However, it is likely that it could have negative impacts on other clients in the clinic. The rationale for this is that utilizing an art-based assessment incorrectly can lead to misdiagnosis which can result in both ineffective and inappropriate treatment.

A legal question could be "if Brown conducts the training, and one of the participants later uses the assessment which results in a negative or harmful treatment outcome, could Brown be held liable since he knows some of the participants may misuse the assessment?" Topics of liability and legal questions are best answered by a lawyer. The most foreseeable answer to this question is yes, if Brown conducts the training, he could be held liable for negative outcomes directly resulting from a colleague's misuse of an art-based assessment.

6.2.3.2 Assistance from the Literature

Consulting literature is another resource and step of the model that provides assistance within the decision-making process. Literature can provide information regarding the latest evidence for best practices in art therapy and advise on what may be the most ethical decision.

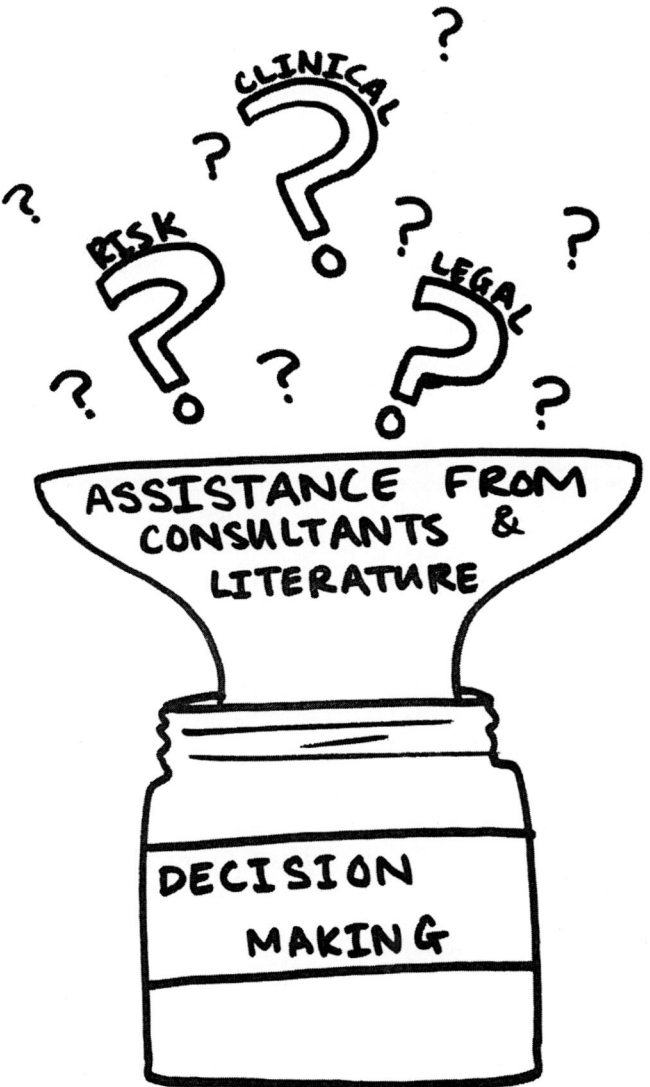

Figure 6.3 Visual representation of assistance from consultants and literature.

Art-based assessments and directives can be administered in an informal or formal process (Deaver, 2016). Formal art therapy assessments, such as the Bird's Nest Drawing, require an understanding and execution of standardized art materials, procedures and directives that are consistent, and knowledge of how to interpret and read ratings on a scoring system when applicable (Deaver, 2016). Research on formal art-based assessments has been ever-expanding and focusing on the proper use of these assessments. These proper uses include (1) the art therapist or professional utilizing the assessment, (2) the method of applying the assessment, and (3) the manner in which the assessment is measured. Factors about the client must also be taken into account for the appropriate use of an art-based assessment. For example, the Bird's Nest Drawing was designed to be utilized with children to assess attachment security and styles, and was not intended to be used with adults. Furthermore, art therapists must also consider cultural and educational factors (Deaver, 2016).

Other recent literature provides guidelines for the proper use of art-based assessments and the intended use of the Bird's Nest Drawing. Research states that while the Bird's Nest Drawing use is encouraged among practicing art therapists and other qualified professionals, the reliability and validity of this assessment is still under research (Yoon et al., 2020). This literature emphasizes the importance of qualified use of assessments and discourages Brown from conducting the art assessment training. This identified need for caution not only applies to Brown's colleagues, but also to Brown for future use of the BND and other assessments where training and competence are necessary for appropriate and safe assessment use.

6.2.4 R-Responsibility/Risk

In this case, the art therapist, Brown faces potential risk from Jane, colleagues, and future clients. To better help this step, Brown chose to adapt the *Draw-a-Person-in-the-Rain* directive (Willis et al., 2010) which is known to assess coping with stress (see Figure 6.4). The drawing here shows Brown, standing in the rain with an inadequate umbrella. The rain or "risk" here is filtering through the tears in the too-small umbrella. Brown is getting covered in rain and needs to find the option with the least risk possible.

6.2.4.1 Option One

If Brown proceeds with option one and refuses to conduct the training, there are a variety of potential risks associated with various parties. The colleagues who are art therapists may end up receiving information and training from an even less reliable source resulting in Brown's colleagues practicing incompetently. This puts Brown in a situation where he will need to determine how to ethically address the incompetent use of assessments by others. Brown also faces risk in the form of a formal reprimand from his supervisor Jane.

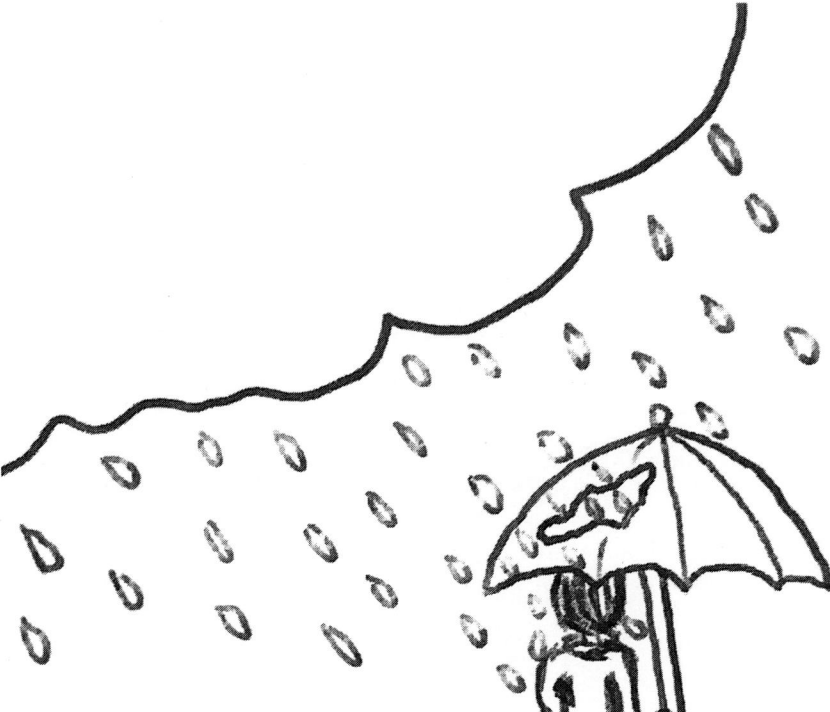

Figure 6.4 Draw-a-person-in-the-rain modified to illustrate the interaction of responsibility and risk.

6.2.4.2 Option Two

If Brown chooses to proceed with training but provides a disclaimer, he faces risk from colleagues and even clients who may be harmed through the inappropriate use of the BND. Specifically, if clinicians in the training decide to misuse the BND, it leaves room for potential mistreatment and harm to clients. However, if the training is approached cautiously and includes disclaimers regarding the limitations for those colleagues, then this risk may be reduced.

6.2.5 T-Take Action

After applying the model and reflecting on the directives created, Brown visually depicts the take action step by utilizing a road drawing directive to represent a crossroad with two paths forward (see Figure 6.5). The drawing represents a relatively smooth road labeled as option two, whereas option one has barriers and various dangerous obstacles. Brown

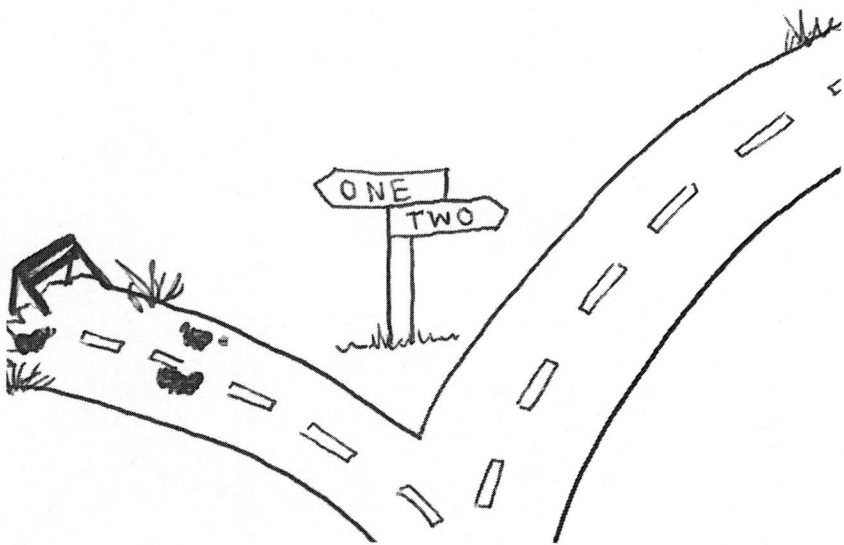

Figure 6.5 Take action step visually represented utilizing a road drawing.

determines that option two where the proceeds with the training but provides a disclaimer seems to be the most ethical approach.

Option two is supported by AATA principles 10.5, 10.8, 8.3, 6.4 and these ensure that services are being used properly and training is implemented to ensure proper use of assessment for the welfare of their clients. These codes also aim to better society and ensure that proper measures are taken for education (American Art Therapy Association, 2013). While this option is discouraged by ATCB code 1.2.3 and AATA Principles 1.0, 3.1 and 3.2, these are outweighed by the high risk and consequences that would come along with them. Option Two has the most positive outcomes on Brown, colleagues, and future clients and is supported by recent literature. In taking action through option two, Brown minimizes risk and ensures that clinicians in the group practice are educated about proper assessment usage.

6.3 Summary of the Main Concerns

Although both the process and product are taken into consideration for art therapy treatment, art-based assessments focus most on the product and content represented in a client's artwork. Art-based assessments may be used for several components in treatment and work with clients but it is important to note that art assessments cannot be utilized for an absolute diagnosis. Indeed, best practices suggest using art-based assessment to increase client insight and abilities. Art therapists should also ensure that no matter what assessment is used, the key component to ethically utilizing art assessments is to have the artwork created in front of the therapist in conjunction with a thorough explanation of the process and content so as to not leave room for therapists to create their own interpretations and narratives.

Art therapists should endeavor to make informed decisions on which art assessments to utilize. Assessment selection should be guided by recent, relevant research as well as the client's background and well-being, which includes the client's cultural background, physical and mental level of functioning, and developmental implications such as age. It is also important to consider the intended use of the assessment, what the assessment is measuring, and the level of reliability and validity of the assessment. Since assessments utilizing the creative process are common in art therapy, the subjective nature of assessment interpretation may leave more room for ethical dilemmas to arise. This further underscores the importance of artwork being created in the presence of the therapist and paired with client input.

Art-based assessments are therapeutic interventions utilized to gather information about the presenting problem(s), diagnosis, and progress toward treatment plan objectives. Assessments allow practitioners to collect information regarding the client's strengths and interactions with certain art mediums and reactions to art directive prompts. In summary, the creative liberty that art therapy provides can be a highly successful form of therapeutic intervention but can also open the door for ethical dilemmas. Consequently, it is important that art-based assessments are utilized in an intentional, valid, reliable, and ethical manner.

6.4 Tips for Avoiding Pitfalls

When using art-based assessments, one tip is to ensure that there is an understanding and level of competence for the art-based assessment selected and administered. It is important to consider the instructions designed for each assessment and to consider which population the assessment is intended for. In addition, it is important to be aware that when utilizing art-based assessments, the artwork must be created in front of the therapist. Furthermore, any explanations and narratives that coincide with artwork or art-based assessment should be explored between the therapist and the client. It is not considered ethical or appropriate to assess or diagnose a client based on the artwork they did not create in a session in front of the art therapist (ATCB, 2021).

Considering the client's developmental level, cultural background, and responses to certain art materials is critical to maintaining ethical and effective practices. As ethical principles and guidelines state, art therapists and other mental health professionals should practice within their scope of competence and incorporate an understanding of the client's culture (American Art Therapy Association, 2013; ATCB, 2021). Finally, consultation is key for navigating ethical dilemmas and provides information and perspective on the situation from other professionals and from literature. When using research as a consultation tool, practitioners should be sure that the literature is recent so as to ensure the information is up to date and relevant.

6.5 Suggested Further Readings

Gilroy, A., Tipple, R., & Brown, C. (2012). *Assessment in art therapy*. London: Routledge.

The book *Assessment in Art Therapy* covers the history and prevalence of assessment used in art therapy. Different cases and approaches to assessments in art therapy are discussed in each chapter. Other chapters include art-based assessments in art therapy and ways to move forward with positive psychology approaches to art assessment. This book provides the reader with foundational information on the approach to directives and art-based assessments in art therapy that can help inform best practices for assessment.

Malchiodi, C. A. (2003), *Handbook of art therapy*. The Guilford Press.

The *Handbook of Art Therapy* provides a comprehensive overview of art therapy, covering a wide range of subjects that provide a thorough guideline for art therapists. This book examines research regarding what can and cannot be determined when viewing artwork made by clients. There are specific chapters that discuss how to approach art-based assessments and what art therapists should be looking out for in client artwork.

References

American Art Therapy Association. (2013). *Ethical principles for art therapists*. https://arttherapy.org/wp-content/uploads/2017/06/Ethical-Principles-for-Art-Therapists.pdf

Art Therapy Credentials Board. (2021). *Code of ethics, conduct, and disciplinary procedures*. https://www.atcb.org/wp-content/uploads/2020/07/ATCB-Code-of-Ethics-Conduct-DisciplinaryProcedures.pdf

Buck, J. N. (1948). The H-T-P test. *Journal of Clinical Psychology*, 4, 151–159. 10.1002/1097-4679(194804)4:2<151::AID-JCLP2270040203>3.0.CO;2-O

Deaver, S. P. (2016). The need for norms in formal art therapy assessment. In D. E. Gussak, & M. L. Rosal (Eds.), *The Wiley handbook of art therapy* (pp. 600–606). Wiley Blackwell.

Harmon-Walker, G., & Kaiser, D. H. (2015). The Bird's Nest Drawing: A study of construct validity and interrater reliability. *The Arts in Psychotherapy*, 42, 1–9. http://doi.org/10.1016/j.aip.2014.12.008

Kaiser, D. H. (1996). Indications of attachment theory in a drawing task. *The Arts in Psychotherapy*, *23*(4), 333–340. 10.1080/07421656.2009.10129312

Kaiser, D. H. (2016). Assessing attachment with the Bird's Nest Drawing (BND). In D. E. Gussak, & M. L. Rosal (Eds.), *The Wiley handbook of art therapy* (pp. 514–523). Wiley Blackwell.

Kaiser, D. H., & Deaver, S. (2009). Assessing attachment with the Bird's Nest Drawing: A review of the research. *Art Therapy*, *26*, 26–33. 10.1080/07421656. 2009.10129312

Kato, D., & Suzuk, M. (2016). Developing a scale to measure total impression of synthetic house-tree-person drawings. *Social Behavior and Personality*, *44*, 19–28. 10.2224/sbp.2016.44.1.19

Kaplan, F. F. (2003). *Art-based assessments*. In C. A. Malchiodi (Ed.), *Handbook of art therapy* (pp. 25–33). The Guilford Press.

Malchiodi, C. A. (2003). *Handbook of art therapy*. The Guilford Press.

McNiff, S. (2012). Art-based methods for art therapy assessment. In A. Gilroy, R. Tipple, & C. Brown (Eds.), *Assessment in art therapy* (pp. 66–80). Routledge/ Taylor & Francis Group.

Naglieri, J. A., McNeish, T. J., & Bardos, A. N. (1991). *Draw-a-person: Screening procedure for emotional disturbance*. ProEd.

Naglieri, J. A., McNeish, T. J., & Achilles, N. (2004). Draw a person test. In Brooke, S. L. (Eds.), *Tools of the trade: A therapist's guide to art therapy assessments* (p. 124). ProEd.

Willis, L. R., Joy, S. P., & Kaiser, D. H. (2010). Draw-a-Person-in-the-Rain as an assessment of stress and coping resources. *The Arts in Psychotherapy*, *37*, 233–239. 10.1016/j.aip.2010.04.009

Yoon, J. Y., Betts, D., & Holttum, S. (2020). The Bird's Nest Drawing and accompanying stories in the assessment of attachment security. *International Journal of Art Therapy*, *25*, 76–87. 10.1080/17454832.2019.1697306

7 Art as a Record: Storage and Exhibition of Client Artwork

Amanda Bezold, Jongwon Melissa Choi, and Jenna Park

Throughout the years in the field of art therapy, there has been debate and controversy on the ethics of client artwork becoming a part of their clinical record, the storage and maintenance of client artwork, and exhibiting artworks created within the context of therapy. Many art therapists in the field have addressed the ethics of storage and exhibition (e.g., Moon & Nolan, 2020; Malchiodi, 2012; Hammond & Gantt, 1998). This has been a recurring topic as revisions were made to the American Art Therapy Association's (American Art Therapy Association, 2013) *Ethical Principles for Art Therapists* and the Art Therapy Credential Board (ATCB, 2021) *Code of Ethics, Conduct, and Disciplinary Procedures* (Malchiodi, 2012; Hammond & Gantt, 1998). In the United States, credentialed art therapists are guided by the codes and principles set forth by both the American Art Therapy Association (2013) and ATCB (2021), which overlap when it comes to record-keeping, storage, and exhibition.

Art therapy ethical codes were created to keep the client's safety and needs primary. From the informed consent process which starts at the beginning of treatment, clients should be made aware of the exact ramifications that delineate how their artwork will be stored, and the kinds of questions that might arise if the artwork is displayed in the office or exhibited in a gallery setting. If a client is a minor, art therapists seek assent from a legal guardian or parent. While informed consent attempts to cover all aspects of therapy, it is still difficult to ascertain the ethical dilemmas that may come up related to storing and exhibiting artwork.

7.1 Art as a Record

The safeguarding of client records is mandatory in the standard of care in therapy (American Art Therapy Association, 2013). Artwork created in a therapeutic setting may contain explicit material which needs to be protected. Therefore, art therapists may include client artwork into a client's record, as outlined by American Art Therapy Association (2013) principle 4.0, which states that artwork is regarded as a form of protected information and property of the client. However, there is strong disagreement about

DOI: 10.4324/9781003175124-7

whether artwork should be placed in the record, as a client's confidentiality may be compromised (Hammond & Gantt, 1998; Moon & Nolan, 2020; Malchiodi, 2012; Rubin, 2011; Spaniol, 1990). Controversially, the institutional policies and procedures of one's workplace oftentimes dictate what happens to client artwork. For example, some settings may require artwork to become a part of a client's record. Sharing client artwork with an interdisciplinary team may be appropriate, especially when containing imagery that suggests suicidal ideation, violent behavior, or psychiatric regression (Hammond & Gantt, 1998). Regardless of practice, American Art Therapy Association (2013) principle 4.7 states that art therapists explain to the client how the artwork will be stored. Typically, this is done at the beginning of treatment in informed consent.

7.2 Storing Artwork

Storage is an important part of maintaining an art therapy space and is a key aspect in protecting sensitive client artwork. Over the years, the accumulation of artwork from sessions may sometimes exceed the amount of storage space available. For example, some art therapists may have limited storage space and should let clients know in the informed consent process that photographs will replace physical records of artwork. Rubin (2011) points out that artwork is an extension of the person, and the way it is handled, stored, and displayed is a sign of respect, demonstrating how the therapist views the client as well.

Some art therapists have suggested creating an art portfolio folder to hold and organize artwork when they first start treatment (Malchiodi, 2012). In this experience, which usually happens in the first session, the client is given the opportunity to learn about art therapy, go over informed consent, and understand the importance of safely storing the artwork for their privacy. If there is any doubt as to whether artwork can be stored in a confidential manner (e.g., a big sculptural art piece or piece that requires time to dry), the client needs to be made aware beforehand (Malchiodi, 2012; Rubin, 2011). If a client does not want their artwork resting on a shelf or seen by others, the therapist should take care to digitally photograph the artwork after the client has given consent, and provide alternative storage or have the client take the artwork with them between sessions.

7.3 Exhibiting Artwork

Lachman-Chapin et al. (1998) ask the question, "Whose needs are being served by showing clients' art?" (p. 235). Not all clients that come into art therapy sessions consider themselves artists, but art therapists encourage all clients to explore materials and the creative process, sometimes leading to the question of displaying artwork (Malchiodi, 2012). The artwork created during the therapeutic process may serve a variety of purposes, but clients are rarely creating artwork for the purpose of exhibition. The amount of therapeutic emphasis oftentimes influences how artwork is perceived by the client and the interest clients have in displaying artwork. Hammond and Gantt (1998) point out for example, that in an adult day care program less emphasis is placed on therapeutic approaches, where participants benefit from the act of art-making but not from a psychotherapeutic exchange. The goals of exhibiting should always align with the goals of therapy and provide a positive impact for the client rather than be used for marketing or exploitation.

7.3.1 Potential Benefits and Risks of Exhibiting Artwork

While there is always potential for unintended consequences for the clients, art therapists throughout the field have pointed out the benefits of exhibiting artwork created over the course of treatment. For example, exhibiting artwork can empower the client, restore dignity, and raise areas of advocacy in mental health awareness (Moon & Nolan, 2020; Malchiodi, 2012; Spaniol, 1990). Exhibitions can also raise questions and add dialogue to the public awareness of mental health issues and the role of art therapy (Kaplan, 2006). In one example, clients processing trauma from miscarriage infertility, and stillbirth were given the opportunity to display artwork and it provided them an opportunity to validate their feelings, as well as receive community support in their healing journey (Andrus, 2020).

In another example, Houpt et al. (2016) discuss the project titled Write for You, which took place with residents in a skilled nursing facility. Members were encouraged weekly to use words, comics, and collages for self-expression in group art therapy, which then culminated into a zine that was distributed and shared with the staff and other community members. Before exhibiting their artwork, precautions were taken in regards to consent forms, and after finding successful feedback from the facility, their artwork was exhibited nationally, touring in different festivals and conferences (Houpt et al., 2016). The zine, titled *Anti-Memoir*, served as a way to share the experience of the older adult, increasing visibility for members as valuable contributors to society, while simultaneously pointing out stereotypes and elevating their voices both inside and outside the nursing home (Houpt et al., 2016).

Rubin (2011) notes that at one time, many art therapists worried that exhibiting or reproducing a client's artwork was a form of exploitation. However, drawing from her own experience, she indicates most individuals have been more than happy to have their work displayed whether in an exhibit or reproduction in a book or calendar (Rubin, 2011). Moving client stories outside of the private realm of therapy into the public also has the potential to be transformative. Throughout recent literature, many authors have alluded to exhibiting artwork in museums or collaborating with local galleries and agencies (Andrus, 2020; Coles & Jury, 2020; Watson et al., 2021). Dejkameh and Shipps (2018) and Watson et al. (2021) describe group art psychotherapy sessions held in museums and the potential for museum-based art therapy to provide resources for individuals to improve their lives.

While there are many benefits of exhibiting client artwork, art therapists have also identified potential risks as well. Some areas of concern are exploiting client artwork versus advocating and appropriately exhibiting artwork (Davis, 2017; Moon & Nolan, 2020; Malchiodi, 2012; Vick, 2011; Spaniol, 1990). For example, artwork hung in a school setting like a hallway, potentially breaches client privacy and opens more discussion amongst peers, teachers, and staff that might not work for the benefit of the client (Knowles, 1996).

7.3.1.1 The Case of Sung

Sung, an art therapist with his own private practice, is about to move his counseling office to a new location. In his current space, he has a meticulously designed storage area that contains all his client artwork, organized by year. It has been close to 10 years since he opened his practice and he has kept all client artwork since then. He has successfully terminated therapy with each client and has kept any artwork the client did not want upon completion.

In preparing for the move, Sung realizes that there is way more than he is able to transfer to his new practice location. Some of the artwork is larger in size (see Figure 7.1) and will be difficult to transfer and store (see Figure 7.2). He wonders if it would be best to begin creating digital representations of the larger artwork pieces. Sung refers to the informed consent that he originally issued to his clients, which states he will maintain artwork for 7 years if the client did not want it after therapy was terminated. The consent details the overall process of the art therapy services provided, the number of treatment sessions, the goals of treatment, and how long the art created during treatment will be stored upon termination. However, the original consent does not indicate what will happen to the artwork if his practice moves locations. The consent also does not include any details regarding the photographic representation of client artwork. At this time, Sung ponders whether it is ethical to dispose of the artwork that is over 7-years-old and make digital copies of the remaining artwork (i.e., less than 7-years-old).

7.3.1.2 Analysis of the Case

Sung is faced with the dilemma of whether or not it is in the clients' best interest to create digital representations of artwork that is under 7-years-old. In order to come to the best ethical decision, Sung considers the ethical codes of the *American Art Therapy Association* (American Art Therapy Association, 2013), and the *Art Therapy Credentials Board* (ATCB, 2021).

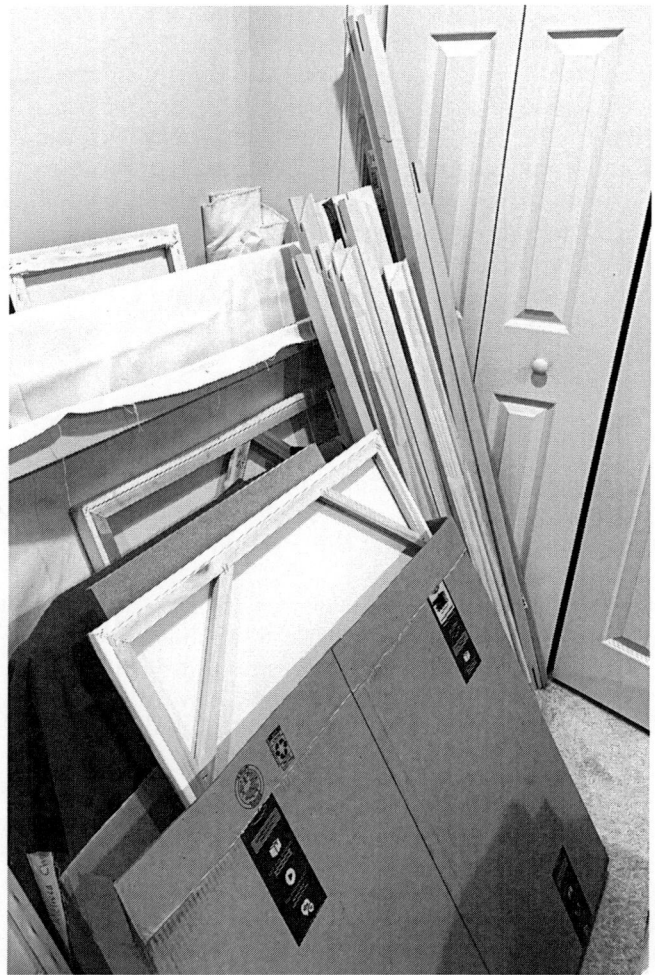

Figure 7.1 Artwork may not always be easily stored, based on size, shape, and weight. Retention must always be considered.

7.4 D-Dilemma

In the case of Sung, there are two viable options. Option One is to make digital representations of client artwork, and Option Two is to not make digital copies and dispose of the pieces he is unable to transfer to his new location. In Figure 7.3, Sung has visually depicted the relevant ethical codes and principles on four continuum lines. The first and second lines show American Art Therapy Association (2013) principles 4.0 and 1.0 and ATCB (2021) codes 2.1.8, 2.1.9, and 2.2.1, with dots that represent

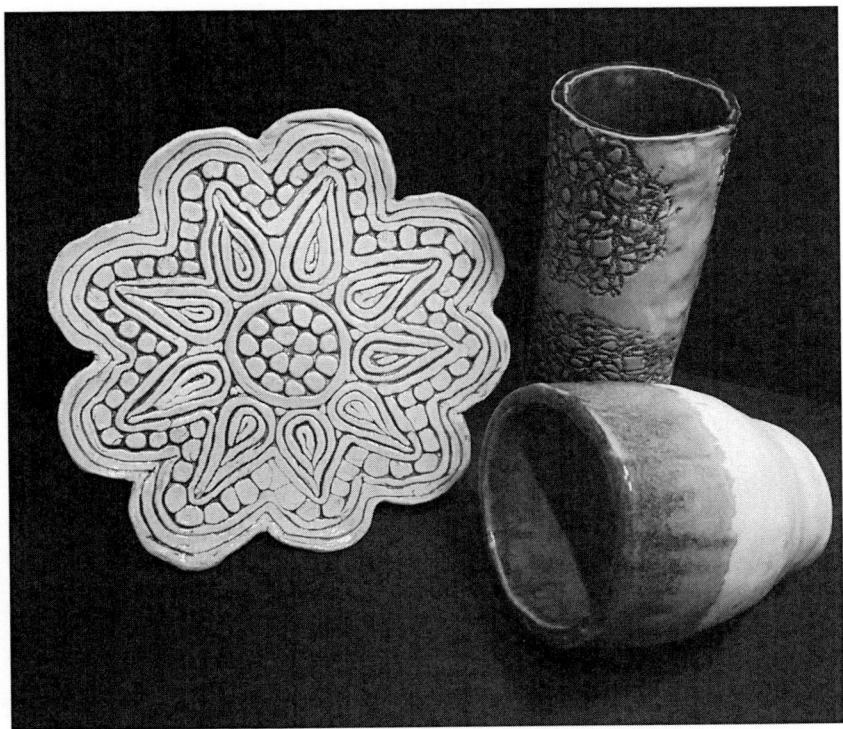

Figure 7.2 Artwork that is three-dimensional, fragile, or heavy may be hard to maintain in a client record.

support for making digital copies of artwork (Option One). The third and fourth lines show American Art Therapy Association (2013) principles 4.7, 4.1.a, and ATCB (2021) code 2.2.3 with the dots closer to the decision of not making digital copies of artwork (Option Two).

7.4.1 Option One: Codes and Principles Supporting Option One

Option One consists of Sung making photographic digital copies of client artworks that are less than 7-years-old. In support of Option One are ethical standards from the American Art Therapy Association (2013) and ATCB (2021). Client access, storage, and retention of artwork are supported by American Art Therapy Association (2013) principle 4.0, which advises art therapists that client artwork may be part of the clinical record and maintained as such. By maintaining digital copies, Sung is avoiding harm to his clients if copies of artwork are needed in the future. Sung also has a responsibility to his clients to protect their welfare, which includes

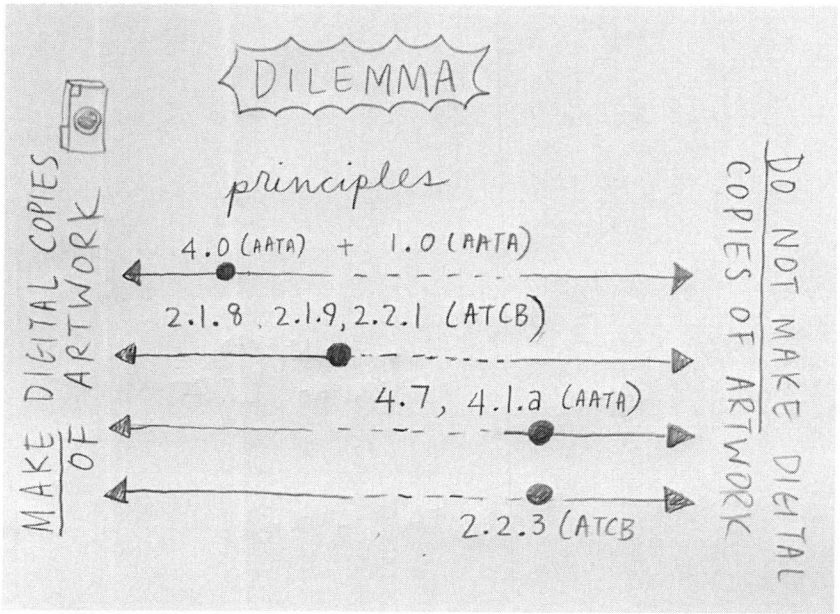

Figure 7.3 AATA and ATCB Ethical principles are depicted on continuum lines as a visual representation of the Dilemma Step.

maintaining adequate records. This also aligns with the American Art Therapy Association (2013) principle 1.0.

In further support of Option One are ATCB (2021) codes 2.1.8, 2.1.9, and 2.2.1. Code 2.1.8 pertains to the preservation of client records for the amount of time devised by federal and state laws of the therapist's jurisdiction (ATCB, 2021). Further, code 2.1.9 ascertains that photographic representation of client artwork may be obtained when appropriate consent is administered and the artwork is difficult to contain under normal circumstances (ATCB, 2021). ATCB (2021) code 2.2.1 also lends support for Option One as this code advises art therapists to consider the cost and benefit ratio of duplicating client artwork through means of photographing. Sung is weighing the costs and benefits of creating digital representations of previous clients' artwork.

7.4.2 Option One: Codes and Principles Discouraging Option One

If Sung decides to create digital representations of the artwork he may be violating ethical codes and principles. American Art Therapy Association (2013) ethical principle 4.1.a discourages this because clients must be notified when the art therapist is maintaining or will maintain copies or photographic representations of artwork. In addition American Art Therapy Association

(2013) principle 4.7 states that clients will be told how their artwork will be stored during treatment as well as how long the artwork will be stored following the termination of treatment. If Sung decides to make digital representations of the accumulated artwork, clients who have not yet been notified of this new storage procedure would need to be advised as well as agree to an updated informed consent. Similarly, ATCB (2021) code 2.2.3 offers provisions against Sung creating a digital representation of his past clients' art. This standard ascertains that the therapist will obtain consent before any photographs of artwork are taken. Since Sung might have difficulty obtaining consent for digitizing client artwork, these principles/codes would discourage the conversion of client artwork to a digital medium for storage purposes.

7.4.3 Option Two: Codes and Principles Supporting Option Two

Although there are ethical standards that provide support for Option One, Option Two must be given similar consideration in order to make a sound ethical determination. Option Two consists of Sung disposing of the artwork he is unable to take to his new practice, rather than creating the digital representations. In support of Option Two is the American Art Therapy Association (2013) aspirational ethical principle of nonmaleficence which discusses avoiding harm or future harm to clients. In creating digital representations without consent Sung may inadvertently cause harm to his previous clients.

Further support for Option Two is provided by the American Art Therapy Association (2013), specifically principle 4.1.a, which states the client must be informed when the art therapist preserves copies or representations of artwork in the client's record. Without obtaining consent, Sung would be in violation of this art therapy principle. Related to this is the American Art Therapy Association (2013) principle 4.7, which advises art therapists to clarify to clients the nature of artwork retention and the manner in which this is done. ATCB (2021) code 2.1.2 advises art therapists to protect confidential information obtained from clients, including artwork and client records, which Sung would be upholding by disposing of the older records.

7.4.4 Option Two: Codes and Principles Discouraging Option Two

Two principles that discourage Option Two are American Art Therapy Association (2013) 2.7 and 4.1, which state that art therapists maintain treatment records during treatment and release artwork to clients when indicated. Likewise, ATCB (2021) code 1.1.15 suggests that art therapists provide access and release records to clients when appropriate. If Sung decides to dispose of artwork, he would be in direct violation of these principles and codes. For example, he would not be able to respond to a client's request for previous artwork due to lack of comprehensive re-cords. In examining the ATCB (2021Art Therapy Credentials Board 2021) codes, Sung would also be in violation of 2.7.1, which specifies artwork must be conserved as devised by state regulations or licensure agreements within the practicing jurisdiction. In disposing of artwork early, Sung may not be upholding the standard to maintain records following treatment termination in accordance with the laws of his jurisdiction.

7.5 O-Outcomes

The various individuals who may be impacted by Sung's ethical decision include Sung, previous clients whose artwork he has maintained, and his current clients. Sung visually depicts the objects and thoughts associated with each option (see Figure 7.4). In the top portion labeled Option One, Sung draws a camera with an arrow pointing to a laptop, implying that digital copies should be made which might be overwhelming. In Option Two, Sung visually depicts throwing artwork out in a waste bin, which may lead to some negative emotions and confusion from previous clients. Throughout the piece, Sung's thoughts are written out to describe the confusing nature of the dilemma.

7.5.1 Option One

It can be surmised that if Sung decides to make photographic re-presentations of the artwork he may feel relieved that he is able to maintain past client's artwork in case it is needed in the future. He will also have established a new procedure within his practice and can apply this to future clients of his new practice. However, Sung may feel over-whelmed in implementing this option, as he would have to contact seven years of previous clients and obtain consent that it is permissible to photograph their work.

Sung's former clients may also be affected by his decision to photograph client artwork. The clients he is contacting may have been in treatment with him many years ago, and he may have difficulty locating them. Contacted clients may react poorly to communication from a former therapist. Further, clients may not remember the artwork they created in treatment and may be confused by Sung's inquiry. It is also possible that a client may request to view their work prior to consenting to the digitization of their artwork, and negative reactions might result from doing so.

Sung's current clients may also be affected by his new procedures. In adapting his informed consent procedures, Sung will also have to obtain updated consent forms from his current clients, and they may be confused as to why these treatment record details were not incorporated in the original consent they received regarding treatment and may question Sung's ability and competency as a therapist.

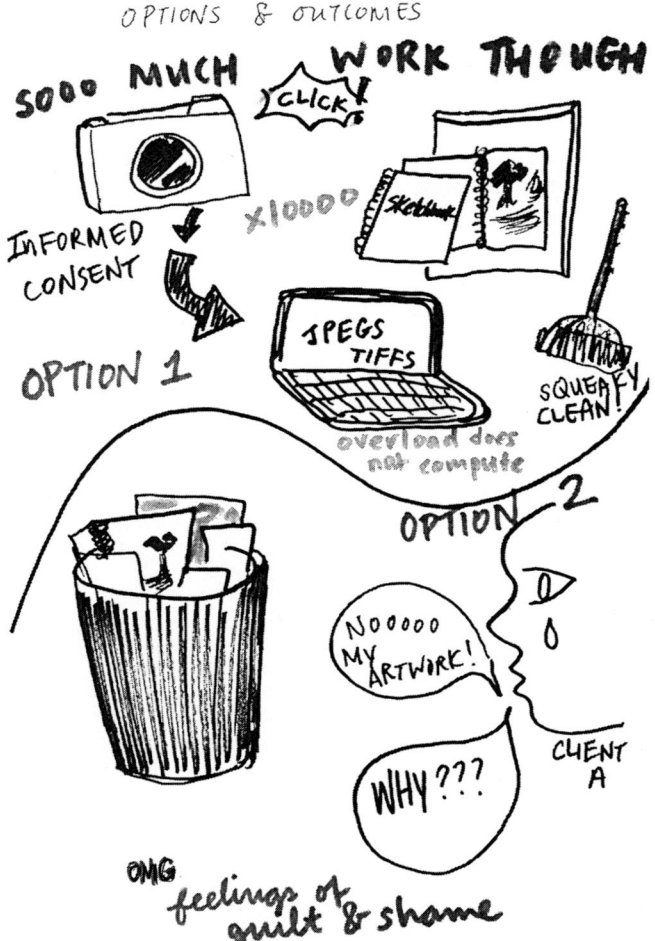

Figure 7.4 Outcomes is represented by objects, images, and words associated with storing and taking photos of artwork.

7.5.2 Option Two

If Sung decides to dispose of artwork, he may have a fresh start at his new practice and be able to keep his current files more organized with the knowledge that art storage space is not unlimited. However, if a prior client were to contact him in the future to obtain files, the record may be incomplete due to missing artwork. This may also inadvertently have a negative impact on clients who are seeking records for new or continued treatment. The artwork being disposed of may be of great importance to clients and/or their new counselors. Clients may feel betrayed by Sung as they had expected the artwork to be maintained for the allotted amount of time originally discussed in the informed consent process.

7.6 A-Assistance

To visually represent the assistance stage, Sung draws himself entering a room filled with questions for consultants and a library of books, which depicts external and internal sources of assistance respectively (see Figure 7.5).

7.6.1 Assistance from Consultants

In order to assist Sung in making the most appropriate ethical decision, he may follow American Art Therapy Association (2013) principle 1.7 by consulting other therapists and supervisors to seek out advice regarding risk management. Sung may want to know, "Have you ever had to condense your client artwork storage? Did you include photographic representations of client artwork in your original informed consent for treatment? Have you had previous clients or other counselors request art records of patients?" Other therapists may have had similar issues in the storage of client artwork and be able to shed some wisdom on Sung's current quandary. A supervisor or colleague may say that to accommodate client requests for records, it is helpful to maintain digital records in order to transcend physical storage limitations. This recommendation from a supervisor lends support for Option One, to create digital copies of artwork, as the records may be irreplaceable and the digital copies will help with storage solutions.

7.6.2 Assistance from the Literature

To gain an additional perspective of the situation, Sung may consult recent literature to help guide his ethical decision. Figure 7.5 further shows the various sources of literature on the left side of the room that Sung uses after consulting with therapists and supervisors. Moon and Nolan (2020) discuss the ethical considerations of client artwork ownership as well as storage procedures and suggest that informed consent documents storage and retention procedures of client artwork. As Moon and Nolan (2020) articulate, the space, cost, and time of storing client records are seldom discussed in the literature. For example, the type of treatment facility may delineate the storage procedures an art therapist must follow. Some therapists may take digital copies of artwork, while other therapists may choose to maintain a physical folder for each client. Most art therapists generally agree that the artwork created within a treatment setting belongs solely to the client they are working with, and therefore it should be up to

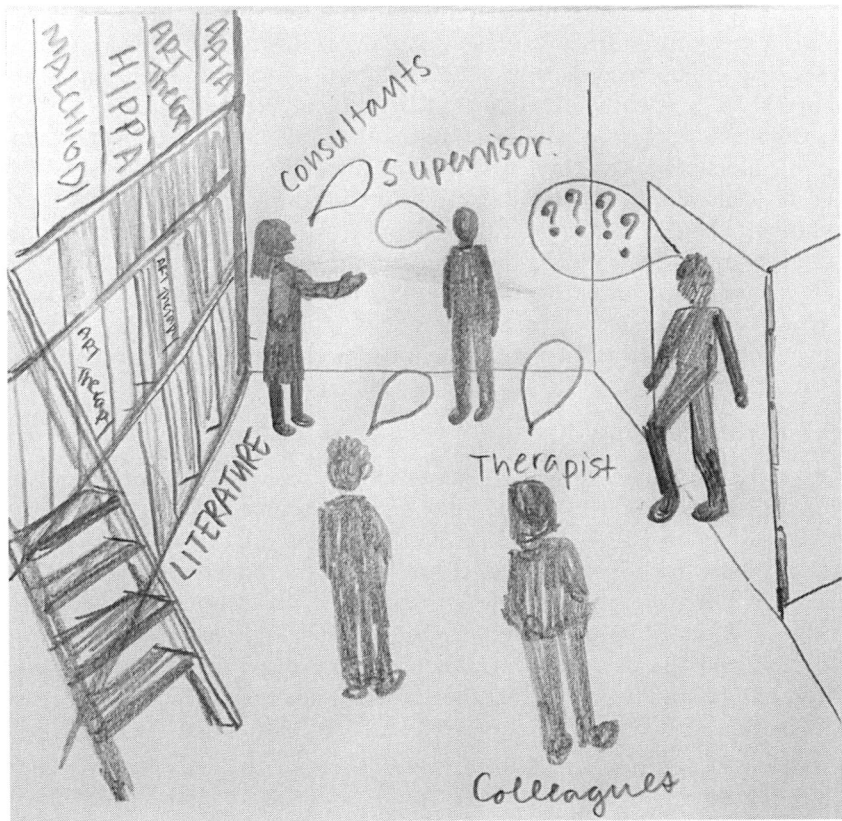

Figure 7.5 A room depicting the assistance step, with both internal and external resources that Sung must consult. He is seen entering a room filled with questions for consultants and a library of books.

the client's discretion to decide what happens to the artwork after therapy is completed; however it is less clear who owns the artwork if it is left behind after termination (Moon & Nolan, 2020). This course suggests that if the artwork belongs to the client, Sung should create digital copies of the work for the clients' potential future use.

As Sung considers the options of creating digital representations of artwork, he may also consider literature noting facilities such as hospitals or mental health centers do not always delineate the nature of the artwork procedures in the original informed consent (ter Maat & Espinola, 2016). In these situations the art therapist must administer a secondary consent detailing these procedures to the client. If digital representations of artwork are to be created, the art therapist must also consider how this data will be stored and the necessary encryption procedures that must be put in place to protect digital copies (ter Maat & Espinola, 2016). Under the Health Insurance Portability and Accountability Act (HIPAA) security rule, safety procedures must be enacted in professional settings to protect sensitive digital records, to further ensure the integrity of electronic record keeping (Centers for Disease Control and Prevention, 2018).

Similarly, Malchiodi (1995) expresses the difficulty with artwork retention, namely photographing artwork and maintaining photographs. It may be difficult for an art therapist to determine what artwork needs to be photographed. Depending on the length of treatment, there may be a plethora of artwork created by the client and the therapist must decide what is important to document (Malchiodi, 1995). In Sung's case, it may be difficult to delineate the artwork that necessitates photographing after 10 years, suggesting that Option Two may be a better choice for older artwork.

7.7 R-Responsibility/Risk

Regardless of which option is selected, Sung is responsible for his clients and must consider risks and liability he may incur. Sung has adapted the Draw-a-Person-in-the-Rain directive (Verinis et al., 1974; Willis et al., 2010). This directive is modified to show risk and management of responsibility as represented by the rain and protection from the rain (Hauck & Ling, 2020). Sung has visualized a large umbrella protecting himself and the client artwork that is to be disposed of from lack of storage (see Figure 7.6). While the artwork may seem disposable because much time has passed, they were created by individuals that he must protect and respect as an ethical counselor.

7.7.1 Option One

If Sung decides to make digital representations of the artwork he may be liable for clients where he is unable to obtain the appropriate consent. While Sung may be upholding his responsibility in maintaining clients' artwork, he may not be adhering to legal aspects of his clinical work nor will he be upholding ethical guidelines to obtain consent for photographing client artwork under American Art Therapy Association (2013) principle 4.2. Consequently Sung may be exposed to legal and/or ethical risk if an investigation or audit were to occur of his client records. However, he would be upholding the American Art Therapy Association (2013) ethical value of nonmaleficence, in avoiding harm that could be caused by not maintaining a form of the records for his previous clients.

7.7.2 Option Two

By disposing of the client's artwork he is unable to transfer to his new practice, Sung may not be fulfilling his responsibility to maintain

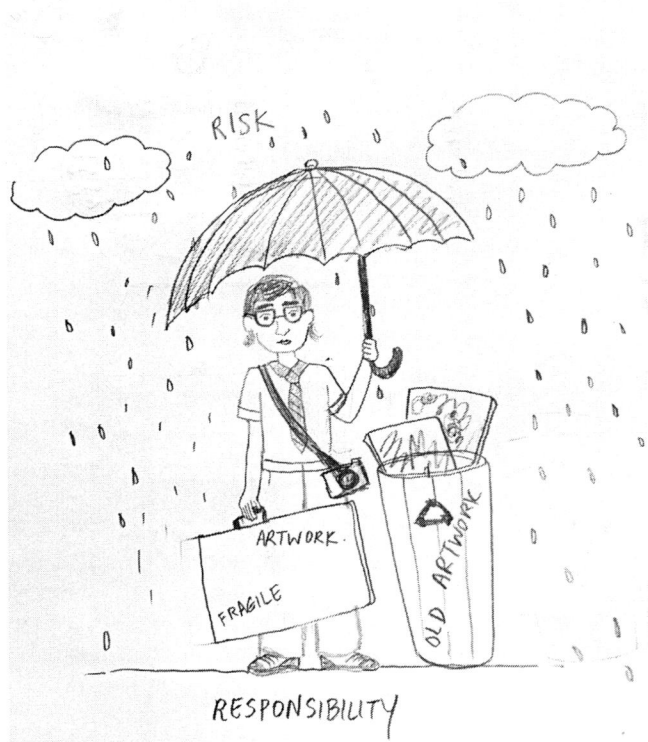

Figure 7.6 Responsibility and risk depicted using the Draw-a-Person-in-the-Rain directive. Sung's umbrella is a metaphor for the protection of risk to old client artwork.

adequate records for his previous clients. If a client requested access to old artwork, Sung may not be able to provide the client with the documents they are seeking. Additionally, Sung may be held liable for not keeping records for the allotted duration of time under his jurisdiction, in accordance with ATCB (2021) code 2.1.8. In choosing ethical decision two, Sung may not be upholding his role as an art therapist or his responsibility to his clients to adequately maintain artwork.

7.8 T-Take Action

After reviewing the various aspects of the situation, Sung's decides on Option One, which involves making digital representations of the artwork and obtaining consent from past clients in order to do so. To visualize coming to his solid decision, Sung draws an orchid plant in his new office (see Figure 7.7). The roots are exposed, similar to the transparency of notifying and obtaining informed consent from past clients. Sung depicts the orchid as having produced several new flowers, which also symbolizes growth and moving forward in his new private practice. In support of this option is the American Art Therapy Association (2013) aspirational ethical principle of nonmaleficence, principles 1.0 and 4.0, and ATCB (2021) codes 2.1.8, 2.1.9, and 2.2.1.

The supervisory advice and the literature lends support for Option One. Although there are additional logistics Sung must consider, the artwork ultimately belongs to the clients who created it in treatment (Moon & Nolan, 2020). By creating digital representations of artwork, Sung is upholding his responsibility to past clients, avoiding undue harm, and decreasing his liability. Although the consent process Sung will have to undertake will be quite lengthy, it is the most ethical option.

7.9 Summary of the Main Concerns

Several concerns are present with regard to the storage and exhibition of client artwork. Art therapists hold the responsibility to be as transparent with their clients as possible, detailing storage and exhibition procedures in informed consent. This responsibility to client artwork is outlined in principles 4.0 and 5.0 (American Art Therapy Association, 2013) and codes 2.1, 2.2, and 2.7 (ATCB, 2021). In storing artwork, art therapists are required to maintain client treatment records and documentation to be consistent with federal, state, and institutional laws and regulations, storing or disposing of records in ways that maintain confidentiality (American Art Therapy Association, 2013; ATCB, 2021).

When faced with an ethical concern on the storage of artwork created in treatment, it is important to involve clients in the decision making process (Walden, 2015). This relates to the aspirational ethical principle of autonomy which is reflected in principle 1.1 (American Art Therapy Association, 2013) and code 1.2.6 (ATCB, 2021), which gives a client the right to control decisions that affect their life, including the choice to display artwork created during sessions.

Moon and Nolan (2020) note that each art therapist needs to decide their stance on ownership, storage, and exhibition and decide how it can coexist with institutional policies and laws. For example, an ethical dilemma that arises within an interdisciplinary treatment team may involve addressing more difficult and complex questions than dilemmas faced by independent practitioners. Furthermore, with an increase in practitioners involved, the chances of confidentiality being compromised increases.

Ethical guidelines are periodically updated, and it's essential that therapists stay up to date with the current American Art Therapy Association (2013) principles and ATCB (2021) codes. This is of particular importance with digitally storing artwork as new technologies

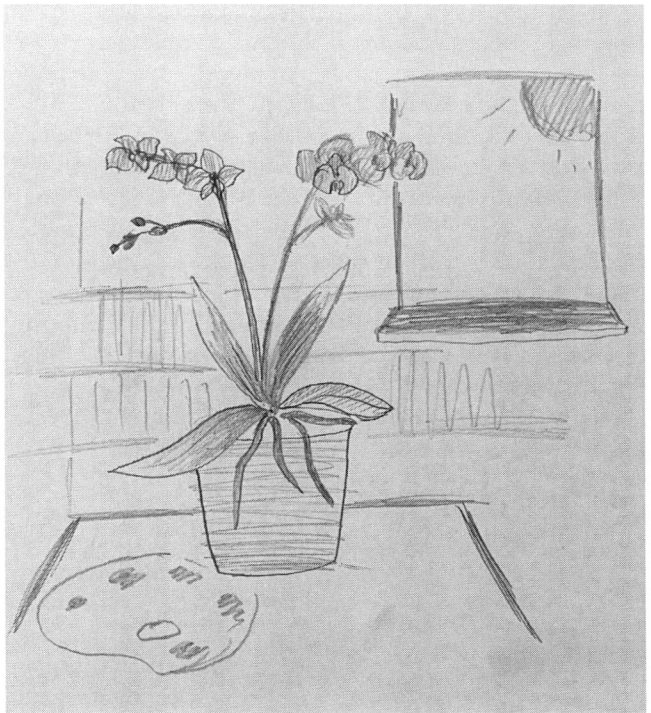

Figure 7.7 Take action step visually represented by the roots and flowers of a sturdy orchid plant in Sung's new office.

advance. Similarly, an art therapist's informed consent also needs to be periodically reviewed to ensure services are being delivered to the highest standards. While an art therapist does their best to include all relevant parties in the informed consent before the start of treatment, issues may arise in regards to storing artwork such as changes in institutional policies, reduction of space in a new office or moving artwork, and receiving proper assent from the parents or legal guardians of minors.

7.10 Tips for Avoiding Pitfalls

Art therapists may implement a number of ethical practices and precautionary measures to avoid encountering ethical challenges in the storage and exhibition of client artwork. As per the American Art Therapy Association (2013) *Ethical Principles for Art Therapists,* art therapists should review with clients how the artwork will be stored, throughout the duration of services and after termination. Transparency regarding artwork storage processes and methods is essential to avoid ethical dilemmas related to retention of original artwork and digital reproductions of the art product. Art therapists can best facilitate client understanding of storage procedures by including comprehensive information regarding artwork storage methods and record retention in the informed consent process (American Art Therapy Association, 2013). Further, including relevant information in both the written informed consent document and in verbal discussion throughout treatment will ensure all parties understand treatment practices. When determining storage methods, art therapists should consider the efficiency, practicality, and privacy implications of all storage solutions.

When utilizing digital record keeping, Art therapists should contemplate the potential benefits and detriments of photographing or otherwise duplicating client artworks, as well as the ramifications of digital storage (ATCB, 2021). Prior to creating digital replicas of client artwork, the art therapist must obtain consent to photograph or otherwise reproduce art products (American Art Therapy Association, 2013). Art therapists have an ethical obligation to inform clients of confidentiality limitations and restrictions (American Art Therapy Association, 2013) and these discussions should extend to digital artwork storage (Alders et al., 2011). Art therapists should be sure to develop a consent form that adequately addresses the basic risks, purposes, and procedures associated with technology use (Choe & Carlton, 2019). While language regarding technology can be as complex as the specifics of technology use itself, informed consent must be worded in a manner consistent with client cognitive abilities and understanding. Digital record keeping should proceed only once informed consent for artwork replication and technology use is obtained and client understanding of storage methods is ensured.

As electronic record-keeping gains popularity, art therapists must ensure digital art records protect client confidentiality. When digital copies of client artwork are produced and maintained, it is advisable that backup files are created and stored on a separate device from the original files (Alders et al., 2011). Practitioners may choose to keep an external hard drive or flash drive to store confidential digital records. By using this storage method, therapists are able to maintain files on a device that can be secured without physical space limitations. If digital art-making is a component of the therapist's practice, the therapist should ensure that electronic art files are not accessible to other clients during device use (Alders et al., 2011).

In the event a client declines to allow photography or digital storage of artwork, art therapists should have an alternative plan for maintaining records of art products. To respect client autonomy and acknowledge the possession of the art by its creator, art therapists may not digitize client artwork if written consent is not provided (American Art Therapy Association, 2013). It is recommended that art therapists work collaboratively with clients to create an artwork storage plan that best meets client needs, standards, and expectations. Alternative plans to ethically store artwork include therapist retention of the original artwork, or include a written description of artwork in the documentation. As space limitations exist, it may be unrealistic for art therapists to retain large quantities of client artwork for extended periods of time and this exemplifies the need for ongoing conversation with clients regarding artwork storage methods (American Art Therapy Association, 2013). It is important for art therapists to maintain records inclusive of client artwork during the course of services to allow ongoing assessment and review of pertinent themes and imagery throughout treatment (Moriya, 2006). As such, while treatment is ongoing, art therapists are responsible for maintaining documentation of client artwork that can be accessible for review throughout the duration of services. Upon culmination of art therapy services, practitioners and clients may collaborate on the ongoing storage of original art products. Clients may retain artwork upon the termination of treatment, alleviating the therapist's responsibility to maintain the art product (American Art Therapy Association, 2013). Art therapists should consider client preferences and discuss practical art product storage methods during the termination process.

With regard to an exhibition of client artwork, art therapists must remain cognizant of ethical obligations and duty to uphold the principle of nonmaleficence. The ethical art therapist facilitates collaborative informed decision-making with the client when determining the appropriateness of publicly displaying artwork (American Art Therapy Association, 2013). When a decision is made to exhibit, the art therapist assists with cultivating an exhibition that promotes the principle of client autonomy. Andrus (2020) notes that it is the responsibility of the art therapist to utilize the sound clinical judgment to assess and determine the appropriateness of the public exhibition of artwork created during the treatment process. In employing sound clinical judgment, art therapists must weigh the potential benefits of the exhibition with possible determinants and consequences (American Art Therapy Association, 2013). Steps to consider before exhibiting client artwork include engaging in an open discussion with the client about the purpose, function, and potential outcomes of the exhibit. While it is important to empower clients to make informed decisions regarding the exhibition of art created during treatment, art therapists should thoroughly address the complexity of displaying art pieces and engage in comprehensive consideration with the client. For example, in planning an exhibition, art therapists should be sure to discuss the specific details including which art to display, appropriate artist identification, exhibition location, and the distribution of profits should artwork be made available for sale (American Art Therapy Association, 2013). In addition to client preference, art therapists should use clinical judgment to assess the necessity of protecting client identity (Andrus, 2020) while also taking steps to ensure client autonomy and uphold the values of fidelity and nonmaleficence.

7.11 Suggested Further Readings

Alders, A., Beck, L., Allen, P., & Mosinski, B. (2011). Technology in art therapy: Ethical challenges. *Journal of the American Art Therapy Association, 28*(4), 165–170. https://doi.org/10.1080/07421656.2011.622683

This reading examines ethical challenges associated with technology use in art therapy practice. The authors explore components of the American Art Therapy Association's ethical guidelines related to digital media use and provide vignettes to illustrate the implications of technology use in various clinical situations. The effects of technology use on the treatment environment, confidentiality, and informed consent and discussed.

Coles, A., & Jury, H. (2020). *Art therapy in museums and galleries: Reframing practice.* Jessica Kingsley Publishers. https://doi.org/10.1080/2 6907240.2021.1890345

This book explores the utilization of museums and gallery spaces as showcases for artwork created during the art therapy treatment process. Case studies and real-world examples are used to exemplify the practicality of displaying art therapy products in these environments. Considerations and benefits of the collaboration between art therapy and art exhibition are explained.

References

Alders, A., Beck, L., Allen, P., & Mosinski, B. (2011). Technology in art therapy: Ethical challenges. *Art Therapy: Journal of the American Art Therapy Association, 28*(4), 165–170. 10.1080/07421656.2011.622683

American Art Therapy Association. (2013). *Ethical principles for art therapists.* https://arttherapy.org/wp-content/uploads/2017/06/Ethical-Principles-for-Art-Therapists.pdf

Andrus, M. (2020). Exhibition and film about miscarriage, infertility, and stillbirth: Art therapy implications. *Art Therapy: Journal of the American Art Therapy Association, 37*(4), 169–176. 10.1080/07421656.2019.1697577

Art Therapy Credentials Board. (2021). *Code of ethics, conduct, and disciplinary procedures.* https://www.atcb.org/wp-content/uploads/2020/07/ATCB-Code-of-Ethics-Conduct-DisciplinaryProcedures.pdf

Centers for Disease Control and Prevention. (2018). *Health insurance portability and accountability act of 1996 (HIPAA).* Centers for Disease Control and Prevention. https://www.cdc.gov/phlp/publications/topic/hipaa.html.

Choe, N. S., & Carlton, N.R. (2019). Behind the screens: Informed consent and digital literacy in art therapy. *Art Therapy: Journal of the American Art Therapy Association, 36*(1), 15–21. 10.1080/07421656.2019.1565060

Coles, A., & Jury, H. (2020). *Art therapy in museums and galleries: Reframing practice.* Jessica Kingsley Publishers.

Davis, T. (2017). Art therapy exhibitions: Exploitation or advocacy? *American Medical Association Journal of Ethics, 19*(1), 98–106. 10.1001/journalofethics. 2017.19.1.imhl1-1701

Dejkameh, M. R., & Shipps, R. (2018). From please touch to *ArtAccess*: The expansion of a museum-based Art Therapy Program. *Art Therapy: Journal of the American Art Therapy Association, 35*(4), 211–217. 10.1080/07421656.2018. 1540821

Hammond, L. C., & Gantt, L. (1998). Using art in counseling: Ethical considerations. *Journal of Counseling and Development, 76*(3), 271–275. 10.1002/ j.1556-6676.1998.tb02542.x

Hauck, J. M., & Ling, T. J. (2020). Applying art therapy directives to ethical-decision making. *Art Therapy: Journal of the American Art Therapy Association, 37*(1), 34–41. 10.1080/07421656.2019.1667669

Houpt, K., Balkin, L.A., Broom, R. H., Roth, A. G., & Selma (2016). Anti-memoir: Creating alternate nursing home narratives through zine making. *Art Therapy: Journal of the American Art Therapy Association, 33*(3), 128–137. 10. 1080/07421656.2016.1199243

Kaplan, F. F. (Ed.). (2006). *Art therapy and social action.* Jessica Kingsley.

Knowles L. P. (1996). Art therapists exhibiting children's art: When, where, and why. *Art Therapy: Journal of the American Art Therapy Association, 13*(3), 205–207. 10.1080/07421656.1996.10759222

Lachman-Chapin, M., Jones, D. L., Sweig, T. L., Cohen, B. M., Semekoski, S. S., & Fleming, M. M. (1998). Connecting with the art world: Expanding beyond the mental health world. *Art Therapy: Journal of the American Art Therapy Association, 15*(4), 233–244. 10.1080/07421656.1989.10759332

Malchiodi, C. A. (1995). Who owns the art? *Art Therapy: Journal of the American Art Therapy Association, 12*(1), 2–3. 10.1080/07421656.1995.10759112

Malchiodi, C. A. (2012). *Handbook of art therapy* (2nd ed.). Guilford Press.

Moon, B.L., & Nolan, E.G. (2020). *Ethical issues in art therapy* (4th ed.). Charles C. Thomas.

Moriya, D. (2006). Ethical issues in school art therapy. *Art Therapy: Journal of the American Art Therapy Association, 23*(2), 59–65. 10.1080/07421656.2006. 10129643

Rubin, J. A. (2011). *The art of art therapy: What every art therapist needs to know* (2nd ed.). Routledge.

Spaniol, S. (1990). Exhibition art by people with mental illness: Issues, process and principles. *Art Therapy: Journal of the American Art Therapy Association, 7*, 70–78. 10.1080/07421656.1990.10758896

ter Maat, M.B. & Espinola, M. (2016). Ethics in art therapy. In D. E. Gussak, & M. L. Rosal (Eds.), *The Wiley handbook of art therapy* (pp. 814–821). John Wiley & Sons.

Verinis, J. S., Lichtenberg, E. F., & Henrich, L. (1974). The draw-a-person-in-the-rain technique: Its relationship to diagnostic category and other personality indicators. *Journal of Clinical Psychology, 30*(3), 407–414. 10.1002/1097-4679 (197407)30:3<407::AID-JCLP2270300358>3.0.CO;2-6

Vick, R. (2011). Ethics on exhibit. *Art Therapy: Journal of the American Art Therapy Association, 28*(4), 152–158. 10.1080/07421656.2011.622698

Walden, S. L. (2015). Inclusion of the client's voice in ethical practice. In I. B. Herhily, & G. Corey (Eds.), *Boundary issues in counseling* (3rd ed., pp. 63–69). American Counseling Association.

Watson, E., Coles, A., & Jury, H. (2021). A space that worked for them: Museum-based art psychotherapy, power dynamics, social inclusion, and autonomy. *International Journal of Art Therapy.* 10.1080/17454832.2020.1866046

Willis, L. R., Joy, S. P., & Kaiser, D. H. (2010). Draw-a-Person-in-the-Rain as an assessment of stress and coping resources. *The Arts in Psychotherapy, 37*(3), 233–239. 10.1016/j.aip.2010.04.009

8 Ethical Multicultural Practice: A Racist Comment in Group Art Therapy

Miki Goerdt

The ethical principles established by the American Art Therapy Association (2013) define multicultural and diversity competence as "the capacity of art therapists to continually acquire multicultural and diversity awareness of and knowledge about cultural diversity with regard to self and others, and to successfully apply these skills in practice with clients (p. 8)." Since the practice of art therapy involves artistic expression, multicultural competency in the profession requires art therapists consider their choice of artistic tools, materials, and environments to be based on their clients' unique backgrounds. While sensitivity to art material and cultural norms is important, multicultural competency requires more than just a checklist of what art supplies to prepare, how to introduce and appreciate traditional/indigenous art forms, and what questions to ask.

As art therapy has been historically practiced from a white, male, Eurocentric view (Jackson, 2020), the impact of race and racism has not been examined closely in art therapy literature until recent years. Race is an element of diversity mentioned in the American Art Therapy Association (AATA)'s Ethical Principles for Art Therapists (2013) and the Art Therapy Credentials Board (ATCB)'s Code of Ethics, Conduct, and Disciplinary Procedures (2021). Without understanding how race affects art therapy practice, an art therapy practitioner would violate the ethical principles addressed by both of the above documents.

Psychotherapy literature on the management of racism expressed by clients mostly involves individual therapy cases (e.g., Bartoli & Pyati, 2009; MacLeod, 2013). Art therapists also need to equip themselves with the understanding of how to apply their multicultural competency related to racialized communication in group work, because art therapists often conduct therapy in a group format. For this reason, a group art therapy setting was selected for this chapter's case vignette. In group art therapy practice, there are additional layers that complicate ethical practice, such as the therapeutic relationship among participants, the participants' racial makeup as well as the group facilitators' racial makeup, and differences in the level of each group facilitator's own racial identity awareness.

DOI: 10.4324/9781003175124-8

8.1 The Case of Sarah and Kaori

Sarah is a White art therapist, and Kaori is an Asian art therapist, who co-own a group practice. Sarah and Kaori co-facilitate an art therapy group for women, focusing on the use of creative expression for emotional wellness. The group consists of ten participants, including those who identify as White, Black, and Latinx. The participants' ages range from 25 and 75 years old. During a recent session, Jane, a 75-year-old White participant, shared her artwork titled "freedom" and explained that recent social uprising movements in the news devalued White people's freedom while honoring Black people's freedom. Jane voiced that she felt discriminated against by the Black Lives Matter movement saying "People don't care about White people, especially an old White woman like me now. Poor Black people just need to work harder. I worked hard all my life. I can't be responsible for their laziness." She explained that she needed to reclaim her freedom through her artwork. Her artwork depicted a blue sky with white clouds in the shape of a mandala. In the center of the mandala was a female figure that appeared much younger than Jane. As Jane spoke, some participants visibly changed their facial expressions. Kaori noticed disturbed looks from several clients, especially participants of color. As the co-therapist, Sarah jumped in and responded with gratitude for Jane's sharing. Sarah then clarified that the group's focus today was about inner peace and emotional wellness, not about what happens in the outside world/society. The group moved on to share other participants' art. After the group, Kaori felt uncomfortable and unsettled with the way that the discussion was handled by Sarah; even though participants clearly had reactions to Jane's comment related to race and age, the group was discouraged from discussing race and social justice issues. Kaori wonders about how to ethically respond to this experience.

8.2 Analysis of the Case

In this situation, there are two important issues to consider. The first is the racist comment made by Jane. The term *racist* is used here to refer to Jane's comment, applying the definition by Kendi (2019), "A racist idea is any idea that suggests one racial group is inferior or superior to another racial group in any way. Racist ideas argue that inferiorities and superiorities of racial groups explain racial inequalities in society" (p. 20). While it is necessary to address Jane's racially charged comment in order to prevent future harm in the group, the dilemma lies in how to clinically and ethically address these concerns in order to facilitate conscious-raising. Specifically, should Kaori address the racist nature of Jane's comment in the group, or outside of the group with Jane privately? The second issue to consider is how to work with Sarah to address the comments in the group, especially in light of Sarah's decision to discourage members from discussing social justice issues during the group. As with any group therapy setting, Kaori and Sarah would need to coordinate their approach as co-facilitators.

8.2.1 D-Dilemma

Kaori has two options. In the first option, Kaori supports Sarah's decision to discourage the discussion of race in the group, and discuss the racist nature of Jane's comment outside of the group privately. In the second option, Kaori and Sarah facilitate a discussion about racism in the group and discuss the racist nature of Jane's comment.

8.2.1.1 Option One: Principles and Codes Supporting Option One

If this is the chosen option, the group refrains from discussing the racist nature of Jane's comment and keeps the social justice discussion out of the group. This option is supported by the American Art Therapy Association (2013)'s aspirational ethical principle of nonmaleficence and the ATCB (2021) code 1.1.1, which says art therapists respect clients' rights and provide services accordingly. These principles and codes support the expectation that Kaori and Sarah be considerate of all clients in the group (including Jane) and honor their rights. This also affirms Sarah's position to avoid discussing race as a group, especially when other participants have not explicitly asked for such a discussion. Likewise, Sarah and Kaori may consider applying ATCB (2021) code 1.2.3 which speaks to competence. Sarah and Kaori may perceive race and social justice as topics to avoid, feeling that they are not competent enough to facilitate or participate in a discussion.

This option is further supported by ATCB (2021) code 1.2.4 which suggests that art therapists strive to promote multicultural competence taking into consideration individuals' identity statuses, as well as AATA principle 7.2 indicating that art therapists should be sensitive to cultural differences and should provide appropriate interventions. Based on Jane's comments, it appears that she was socialized by the dominant White culture. By not discussing racism and the racist nature of Jane's comment in the group shows Sarah and Kaori's sensitivity to Jane's culture. As a White individual, Jane may not have been exposed to the race-related discussion as much as individuals of color. Naming the racist nature of her comment in the group setting may cause shame in her or make her defensive. Such reactions carve out her willingness to examine the lack of awareness over her actions. It is also important to show sensitivity to Jane's generational culture. Jane is in her 70s, which suggests her young and mid-adult years were influenced by the drug war policies of the 1970s and the promotion of colorblindness as a concept. Given that her generational culture makes Jane more prone to making racist comments, these codes and principles point Kaori and Sarah to the possibility that naming Jane's racist comment in the group setting may cause more harm than discussing it privately.

8.2.1.2 Option One: Principles and Codes Discouraging Option One

While there are principles and codes that support Option One, there are also principles and codes that discourage keeping the discussion outside of the group. For example, American Art Therapy Association (2013) principle 7.5 suggests that art therapists show sensitivity to responses from group members generated from their cultural differences. By keeping the discussion outside of the group, Sarah and Kaori would not be able to create space for other participants to voice their opinions. The art therapists also would miss the chance to gain information from Jane directly regarding her cultural view, a stance supported by American Art Therapy Association (2013) principle 7.6. Additionally, countering ATCB (2021) code 1.2.3, it should be noted that art therapists can only achieve cultural competency by engaging in dialogue. Race talk often risks intense emotions and misunderstanding, for both White individuals and people of color (Sue, 2015). Discussions of social justice and race for most people rarely impart feelings of confidence and comfort. Although methods of conducting race talk can vary, waiting to become competent to address race and social justice with clients should not be a barrier to these discussions.

8.2.1.3 Option Two: Principles and Codes Supporting Option Two

The second option for Kaori is to facilitate a discussion about racism in the group alongside Sarah. Such a discussion would include, and most likely start with identifying the racist nature of Jane's comment. This option is supported by the American Art Therapy Association (2013) principle 1.1 "Art therapists respect the rights of clients to make decisions and assist them in understanding the consequences of these decisions" (p. 3). Some participants in the group expressed negative reactions to Jane's racist comment non-verbally. This principle holds Kaori and Sarah accountable for respecting Jane's rights as well as facilitating Jane's understanding of the negative impact of her comments.

American Art Therapy Association (2013) principles 7.1, 7.4, and 7.5, as well as ATCB (2021) code 1.2.5 discuss multicultural competence and also support Option Two as a culturally relevant intervention. Principle 7.1. states that art therapists should not engage in discriminatory actions (American Art Therapy Association, 2013). Although the art therapists, in this case, did not make the racially charged comment, it is likely their silence and avoidance of race talk in the group setting may contribute to future discriminatory actions in the group and the larger society. In other words, Sarah and Kaori may indirectly promote discriminatory actions unless they named Jane's comment as racist. Given the group includes participants of color, sensitivity to their racial backgrounds and oppression requires Sarah and Kaori to understand racial trauma and the impacts of racism. Racism negatively affects the psychological and physiological states of people of color (Alvarez et al., 2016). If Kaori and Sarah are to demonstrate sensitivity to participants and their racial backgrounds, they must point out the racist nature of Jane's comment and facilitate a discussion of racism.

American Art Therapy Association (2013) principle 7.7 points out the need for art therapists to be aware of an additional ethics guide: *the American Art Therapy Association's Art Therapy Multicultural and Diversity Competencies* (American Art Therapy Association, 2011). This guide demands art therapists gain an understanding of discriminatory practices such as racism as well as sociopolitical issues that affect clients' lives and further supports Kaori and Sarah to be proactive about addressing racism during the group session.

American Art Therapy Association (2013) principle 7.3 explaining that art therapists should be mindful of how their beliefs affect their interventions. Sarah used diversion as her intervention to ignore the racist nature of Jane's comment and discourage discussions about racism. By not being a bystander and addressing Sarah's diversion intervention, Kaori upholds the American Art Therapy Association (2013) aspirational ethical principle of justice. It is necessary that Sarah reflects on the reasoning behind her response and its impact on her clients. Indeed, American Art Therapy Association (2013) principle 10.5 holds art therapists accountable for building a better community and society. To this end, Kaori can address social justice issues in the most ethical and clinically appropriate manner possible. This includes addressing the comments with the group as well as suggesting Sarah seek culturally sensitive supervision to understand social justice issues which is consistent with principle 7.6 (American Art Therapy Association, 2013).

8.2.1.4 Option Two: Principles and Codes Discouraging Option Two

ATCB (2021) codes 1.1.1. and 1.2.4 discourage Option Two by focusing respect for Jane's individual rights and showing sensitivity to her cultural beliefs based on her intersectional identities. In addition, American Art Therapy Association (2013) principle 7.2 states that art therapists must make an effort to learn the different belief systems of all of their clients rather than focusing on marginalized clients only.

To help process the dilemma step, two illustrations were created (see Figure 8.1). One illustration depicts the first option as if the group participants were encapsulated in a box and a bubble. Both layers protect

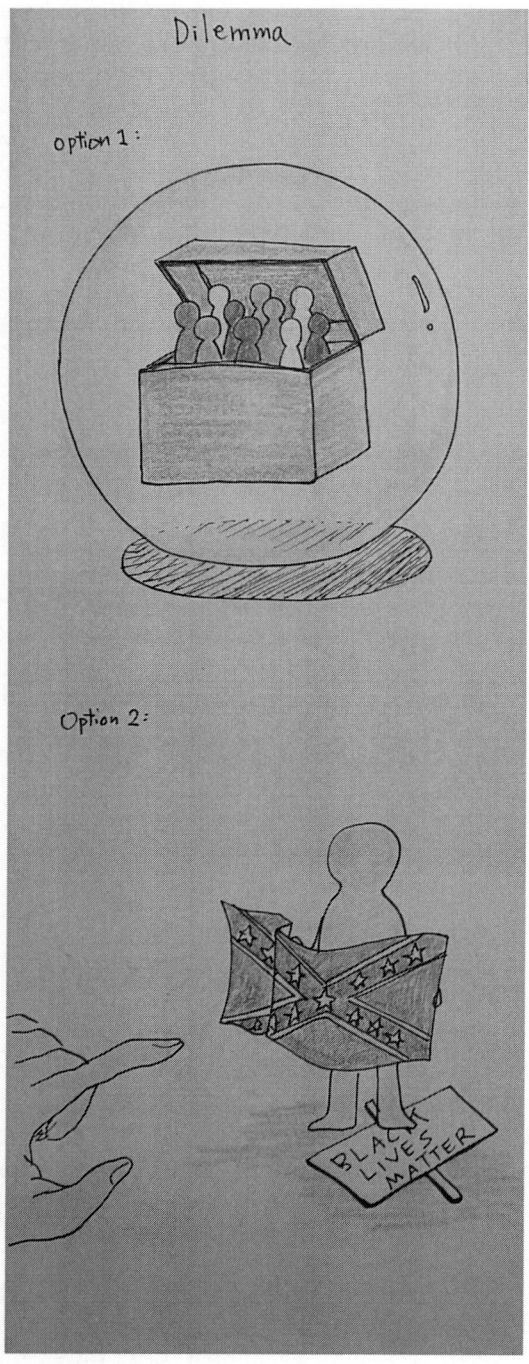

Figure 8.1 Option one is described as placing the group in a bubble, away from the society's influence. Option two is depicted as a finger pointing at Jane.

group participants but also isolate them from the outside world. The other illustration depicts the second option where one of the therapists' fingers is pointing at Jane who is holding a confederate flag and stepping on a Black Lives Matter plaque. Jane displayed no emotion and appeared unaware of the meanings that her actions create.

8.2.2 O-Outcomes

8.2.2.1 Option One

Option One allows Kaori and Sarah to avoid putting Jane on the spot. This also avoids the discomfort of engaging in a discussion over an emotionally charged topic, which could result in a positive outcome for other participants. Specifically, participants of color may already experience exhaustion due to the frequent need to discuss racism and advocate for themselves in their daily lives; discussing Jane's comment could be yet another occasion that they need to deal with.

However, Option One may negatively rupture the sense of safety other participants feel. By not addressing Jane's racist comment in the group, participants (especially participants of color) may feel violated, misunderstood, and re-traumatized. This reduced sense of safety may also result in a reduction of trust participants feel towards the art therapists and group members. This reduction of trust may be experienced differently by Sarah and Kaori due to the difference in their racial backgrounds. Kaori is a person of color and other participants of color may see Kaori as "the other" or "White-washed" when Kaori avoids discussing the racist nature of Jane's comment. With regard to Sarah, participants' expectation of her to identify a racist remark may already be lower because Sarah is White. For this reason, the option of discouraging social justice discussions may cost Kaori more.

Option One also denies Jane an opportunity to gain insight into the negative impact of her comment. A group therapy setting is a place to practice social skills and communication strategies; this is based on the understanding that what happens in the group is a snapshot of what happens in the larger society. Jane may not be aware of the pain her comment inflicts on other participants, and her lack of insight may make others distance themselves from her. This option also eliminates Jane's chance to explore the psychological needs implied by her comment; both racism and ageism bring a sense of powerlessness to those who experience them. It may be that Jane was trying to cope with ageism by inflicting racism onto others, making her feel more empowered. Discouraging discussion of social justice issues may take away her opportunity to more deeply explore her own needs and push her further away from the purpose of this particular group, which is to explore emotional wellness.

In Option One, Sarah and Kaori may privately address Jane's comment with her. From a theoretical perspective, Jane appears to be in the reintegration stage of the White Racial Identity Model (Helms, 2008) characterized by blaming the victim of racism. With this in mind, a private discussion may not prepare her to let go of her belief. According to Helms (2008), Jane would need to either experience "a catastrophic event or a series of personal encounters that the person can no longer ignore" (p. 32). Unlike ongoing discussions of social justice issues in the group setting, a private discussion would most likely fall short as a vehicle for Jane to move forward from the reintegration stage to the pseudo-independence stage, which is the beginning of nonracist White identity development. Even if Sarah and Kaori's private discussion with Jane creates some awareness, the impact of her comment would remain in the group, demanding a repair. She also would lose a chance to be a part of an authentic dialogue and connect with others in the group.

8.2.2.2 Option Two

A negative outcome from Option Two would be that Jane might feel invalidated and alienate herself from the group process. Likewise, group members may experience feelings of discomfort. It is inevitable that the art therapists, Jane, and other participants would experience a range of emotions, including anger, stress, anxiety, sadness, and hurt. The discussion itself may be stressful and traumatizing for all participants, and there may not be a resolution reached at the end of the discussion.

Kaori may also be negatively impacted in Option Two. Since Sarah discouraged the discussion of race, Kaori would have to initiate a conversation with Sarah about the need to discuss social justice issues in order for them to be aligned as group leaders. If Sarah is not well versed in the issues of racism and oppression, Kaori would need to educate Sarah. The act of educating White individuals about racism is painful and exhausting for individuals of color (Oulo, 2018). The less investigation and learning Sarah has done for her racial identity development and cultural competency, the more of an emotional burden Kaori would bear.

There are several potentially positive outcomes of Option Two. First, discussing racism and the nature of Jane's racist comment would promote open communication and authenticity in this group. Corey (2000) asserts that dealing with a conflict in a group setting contributes to building a group norm of accepting negative expressions and thus a deeper level of work. Corey (2000) asserts that allowing conflict empowers participants to take greater risks in therapeutic work.

Second, witnessing others' willingness to take a risk and discuss a difficult topic like race with authenticity can help build trust and a sense of safety between the art therapists and group participants, as well as among participants themselves. Naming the racist nature of Jane's comment in the group discussion would provide validation for some participants. With regard to trust-building, Sarah is at disadvantage in the eyes of some participants of color due to the fact that her racial group has been the oppressor in the larger society. Sarah's Whiteness may make some participants of color feel skeptical of her as a trustworthy provider. Given this background, Sarah's participation in a social justice discussion would positively contribute to building trust with participants.

Third, a discussion of racism may contribute to participants' learning of or attainment of life skills to combat racism. For example, some participants may practice assertiveness to empower themselves, while others may learn how to name racist actions. While the specific skills may differ based on participants' racial identity development, this option would result in a practice of tolerating difficult emotions during a conversation with others. This skill advances social justice as well as maintains healthy relationships with others.

Lastly, the discussion of racism and the impact of Jane's comment provide Jane a chance to gain awareness of her actions and its impact. If Jane is able to examine her thought process by participating in the discussion, there is a possibility that she would make significant progress in her therapeutic process.

As both options were explored through drawing (see Figure 8.2), the core differences between two options became noticeable. The drawing for Option One shows Jane on a pedestal, making other participants feel less important; Kaori and Sarah appear as bystanders without much involvement. The drawing for Option Two shows everyone in the circle, including the therapists. The speech bubbles are in different colors to signify the group members' various opinions. The second drawing shows much more group cohesiveness and inclusivity.

8.2.3 A-Assistance

The dilemmas related to this case vignette are ethical and clinical in nature. The ethical dilemma exists in how Kaori interprets and applies the principles and codes of AATA and ATCB to uphold multicultural competency. Clinically, Kaori's actions would have impacts on the psychological status of all group participants and the therapeutic relationships between the art therapists and group participants. In order to balance ethical obligations with clinical care for group participants, the main question to ponder is what clinical factors would determine the appropriateness of discussing social justice issues in group art therapy. A second question is how to facilitate a discussion on racism in the given

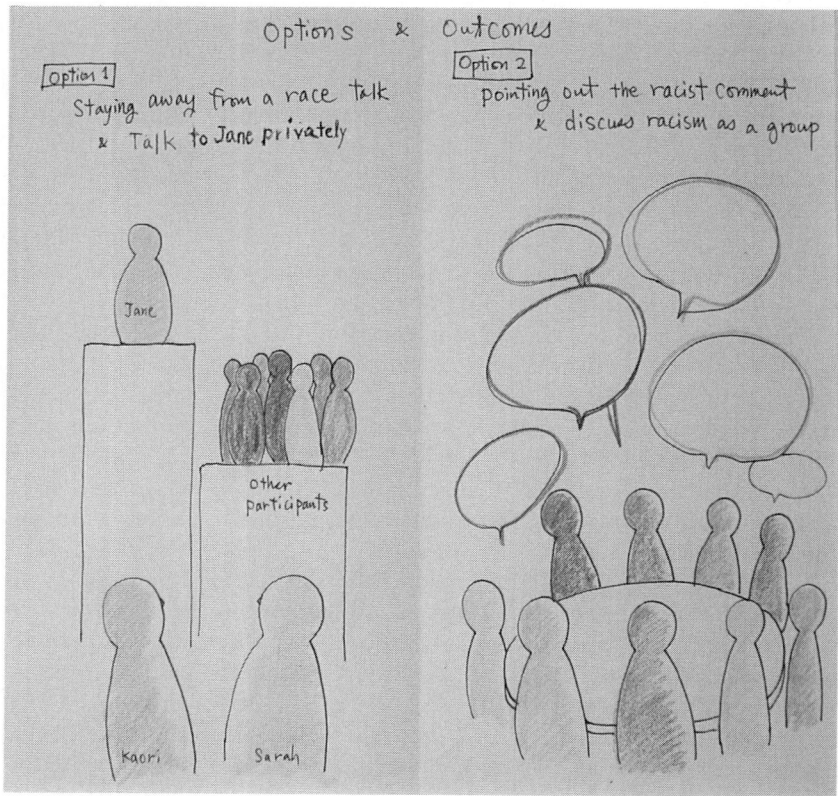

Figure 8.2 Option one depicts Jane being valued more than other group participants. Option two depicts a group discussion.

context of this case, if it is deemed ethically and clinically appropriate to facilitate such a discussion.

8.2.3.1 Assistance from Consultants

Lindsey Vance is one of the leading experts in multicultural art therapy and racial healing. In a consultation about the case (personal communication, February 28, 2021), she pointed out several factors that would determine art therapists' course of action for a racially charged comment in group settings.

First, with regard to the reactions of the group, Vance described how much an acknowledgment of racially charged comments is important especially for participants of color because any lack of action on the art therapists' end would most likely contribute to mistrust between the art therapists and group participants of color. Such an acknowledgment would be necessary even if the group does not have time to fully process the racially charged comment or if they do not come to an agreement. Naming the discomfort created by the comment would likely pave the way for later discussions related to race if participants wish to talk about it in the future.

Next, it is important for the art therapist to assess the group development. The art therapists' actions would also depend on where the group is in terms of group development. How long have group participants known each other? How much trust has been built among participants? How safe do they feel in the group and with the art therapists? If the group was meeting for the first time, the art therapists might not move forward with an in-depth discussion about race after making an acknowledgment. On the other hand, if the art therapists perceive cohesiveness among group participants, the participants may be ready to handle the discomfort associated with an emotional topic like racism.

Third, art therapists should examine what kind of role they play in the group. Some art therapists would choose to stick strictly to a facilitator's role without much self-disclosure. Others would take on a more participatory role. For therapists with the latter style, it is natural for them to share their own reactions to a racially charged comment by a participant in order to open up discussions.

Next, the readiness of each group participant and the group as a whole to explore racial identities should be considered. How much self-exploration has each participant done so far on their own? How much awareness do they have of their lived experience as a racial being, not just what they read in books about their race? What does their own race mean to them? It is also important to take into consideration how much exploration has been done as a group in this area. The group can go more in-depth without sacrificing safety and trust if they have explored this area previously. If they haven't, the art therapists may touch on the topic but not open a full exposure and exploration, out of a concern to prevent harm by asking participants to process what they're not yet ready to process. Should this be the case, Vance recommends the art therapists keep inviting participants back to the discussion and exploration of race in a gradual process.

Finally, it will be important to assess the needs of the group. Vance shared her principle that the group belongs to the group participants. The participants decide what should be discussed in the group, how much to discuss, and the goals of the group. After an initial acknowledgment of the discomfort caused by a racist comment, art therapists can follow the group participants' lead in order to meet their needs. Do participants want to talk about the comment they just witnessed? Or would they rather move on and spend time on something else? Both the art therapists and the participants can view the group session as a ground on which to practice managing similar challenges in the larger society. What do participants need to practice if they recognize that they all live in a racialized society where divisions are so visible? How do they want to contribute to building the society that they envision for themselves?

In particular, to the case, Vance also pointed out the importance of defining emotional wellness. Vance noted that people of color often have more holistic perceptions of emotional wellness, where societal influences are taken into consideration. On the other hand, the dominant culture's perspective on emotional wellness appears to focus on one's internal state and sense of self. Sarah and Kaori need to come to a common understanding of how they define emotional wellness. Vance also suggested the use of cultural humility as a concept to introduce to participants, as well as using group art-making as a way to raise awareness of the influences of race and explore ways to come together with others.

The case was also brought up for a consultation at a local peer supervision group (personal communication, February 28, 2021). This group consists of a psychologist, two social workers, and one dance/movement therapist, in addition to the art therapist/author. This peer group believed that an acknowledgment of Jane's racially charged comment would communicate to group participants that Sarah and Kaori are aware of the racial dynamics at play and are willing to hold space for race-related discussions.

The peer supervision group identified several different approaches that may be helpful in facilitating discussion. First, the therapists' self-disclosure can be used as a tool; Sarah and Kaori can disclose their feelings about Jane's comment as a starting point to facilitate a group discussion. The therapists may experience countertransference as they hear Jane's comment. If they assess their countertransference as helping to increase participants' self-awareness, the therapists may choose to share them with group participants. Disclosing the therapist's reactions calls participants' attention to the moment of discomfort, and this act facilitates participants' introspection into their own reactions to that moment. Introspection can include examining somatic experiences provoked by the comment. Therapists' sharing can be done in a varied degree of articulation based on what benefits participants the most. For example, therapists can share a general sense of discomfort in reaction to Jane's comment, or they may name the racially charged nature of Jane's comment as the specific factor behind the therapists' discomfort.

The peer supervision group also identified the need to clarify the purpose of the group. Since this group is already composed, there can be a discussion to clarify the purpose and goals of the group. If this group was meant to be a mixed-race group, it may be beneficial to have a disclaimer prior to the start of the next group session that some culture-related discomfort may arise during the discussions due to the nature of the group process.

The peer supervision group also discussed clarifying the expectations by having Sarah and Kaori acknowledge the reality that a discussion on race and racism can be uncomfortable and extend the discussion beyond a single session. Participants should expect that people come into groups with various feelings about race and racism, much like in the larger society outside of the group. It would also be helpful to clarify that the purpose of such a discussion is not to decide who is right or wrong. Rather, the discussion can be a place for all participants to consider the concept of the "intent vs. impact" of one's comments, to increase their awareness of the patterns of their own behaviors in and out of group sessions, to explore what brings them the most healing, and to articulate what support they need as a group to achieve the group's goal.

Next, the supervision group pointed out the importance of therapists creating a safe environment to discuss uncomfortable topics such as race. Participants can settle together on group rules that foster safety and trust. What would make them more comfortable to share their thoughts about social justice issues? The group can also identify what makes interactions healthy vs. unhealthy.

Finally, therapists can make a connection between experiences of other "-isms" and racism; When group participants can connect their experiences of other "-isms," such as sexism, they may be able to cultivate their understanding of racism. Jane in particular may cultivate empathy and understanding when she makes connections between ageism and racism. With the therapists, Jane can explore, without using terms such as racism and ageism, if such labels are off-putting. The peer supervision group also suggested that race be mentioned specifically as a factor in Jane's comment before the therapists use this approach, due to the possibility that maintaining silence about race would discourage candid communications about race in the group.

The peer supervision group acknowledged the need to be mindful of time management. Sarah and Kaori could easily spend much of the group time on increasing Jane's self-awareness of her racial identity development. However, this may send the message to other group members that soothing White individuals is the group's priority. It is also worth noting that this particular wellness group was facilitated at a group practice setting, where participants were not mandated to attend. Participants would likely make a decision about their attendance for subsequent sessions based on their experience of the last session. From this perspective, the heavy focus on Jane's needs in this group may cost more than the benefit, as some participants may not return. As an alternative, Sarah or Kaori can offer Jane support outside of the group time for further processing of her individual needs, in addition to acknowledging the discomfort Jane's comment caused and leading social justice discussion.

Sarah's racial identity development was another factor the peer supervision group considered. If Sarah has not explored her own racial identity and its impact on others, it is imperative that she spend time on such an exploration. It would be beneficial for Sarah to facilitate a discussion on race, instead of making Kaori take the lead. The peer support group recommended this because Sarah's act of re-introducing the race-related topic would contribute to rebuilding lost trust with participants. If Sarah feels she lacks the experience to facilitate the discussion, it would be helpful for Sarah to acknowledge race as an important topic and participate in the dialogue facilitated by Kaori. The assumption that a therapist of color would be more capable and comfortable leading discussions of social justice can be untrue and burdensome, and thus Sarah should take Kaori's comfort level with leading such a discussion into consideration.

Both consultations pointed out the importance of acknowledging race as the issue in Jane's comment in the group. Both consultation groups also recommended clarifying the purpose of the group by defining emotional wellness together with group participants. Key factors mentioned in both consultation groups, such as creating a sense of safety and assessing the group's needs, appear to be important for any group setting. It was very clear that such basic group facilitation strategies cannot be effectively implemented unless the therapists have awareness of the racial dynamics in the group and knowledge of racial identity development for participants and for themselves.

8.2.3.2 Assistance from Literature

Ratts et al. (2010) assert that regardless of therapists' intentions, group work that ignores the impact of societal oppression promotes and maintains oppression. In aiming for social justice as a goal and process, Ratts et al. (2010) suggest group leaders create an affirming group atmosphere, where participants actively engage in decision making. Ratts et al. (2010) recommend the Dimensions of Social Justice Model for understanding the degree to which social justice is incorporated within group work. This model is developmental and groups can go back and forth between dimensions. Therapists guide groups to ultimately advocate for themselves, through increased awareness of the social, political, and historical roots of their lived experiences.

Burnes and Ross (2010) hold the view that group work mirrors the reality of the larger society, including social injustice and that this must be acknowledged in the group process. They advise group therapists to immediately process an oppressive comment made by a group participant and recommend weaving social justice work into the group work with the following methods: (1) intentionally composing a group of participants with diverse backgrounds and the ability to be welcoming of all other participants, (2) conducting a pre-screening session before the first session to assess the capacity of each client to discuss oppression in a group setting, (3) viewing the roles that group participants play in the therapeutic setting (e.g., a scapegoat) with an understanding of the roles they play in the larger society based on the oppression and privilege they experience, and (4) using structured activities/exercises to raise participants' awareness of oppression, privilege, and power in a respectful and supportive environment (Burnes & Ross, 2010).

Similarly, Potash (2018) asserts that social justice concerns can be discussed with clients without compromising the ethical principles of nondiscrimination (American Art Therapy Association, 2013, Principle 7.1). "Art therapists can challenge clients and allow themselves to be contested while always maintaining the integrity of the professional relationship (Potash, 2018, p. 206)." Using a case example of his conversation with Black youths at an open art studio, Potash states that discussions about social justice and the impact of discrimination are necessary for establishing a therapeutic alliances. In addition, Potash (2018) addresses the intricacy of discussing racial matters with colleagues and encourages the act of naming as a strategy in order to raise the colleague's awareness and promote change, rather than shaming or calling the colleague out, which could erode trust. These first three sources lend evidence for Option Two.

Conversely, Bartoli and Pyati (2009) caution that it may not be appropriate to assume the necessity of race talk in all therapy sessions. They suggest the following five steps to determine appropriate occasions in which to address a client's racially charged comment: (1) consider the influence of cultural and institutional racism imbedded in the client's thought process; (2) consider how the client benefits from using the beliefs inserted by the cultural or institutional racism in order to cope with their challenges in life; (3) explore the meaning of the client's racially charged comment in the context of the racial composition of the therapeutic relationship; (4) consider the therapist's own motivation to express their views about race to clients in order to make sure the therapist's action leads to addressing the needs of the client; and (5) consider the overall course of treatment and the client's racial identity development status when determining the times to challenge the client's racially charged comment. If therapists deem the client's comment unrelated to the treatment goal, Bartoli and Pyati (2009) suggest that the therapists affirm the client's experience but not validate the content of misconceptions based on racism and prejudice.

Lastly, a racially charged comment addressed by a White therapist may impact the client differently than it might when a therapist of color addresses it. Bartoli and Pyati (2009) speculate that a white client would be less defensive if a white therapist addressed the issue. Jane's response may be different if Sarah is the one naming the racist nature of the comment instead of Kaori; this lends support for Sarah to facilitate the discussion instead of Kaori.

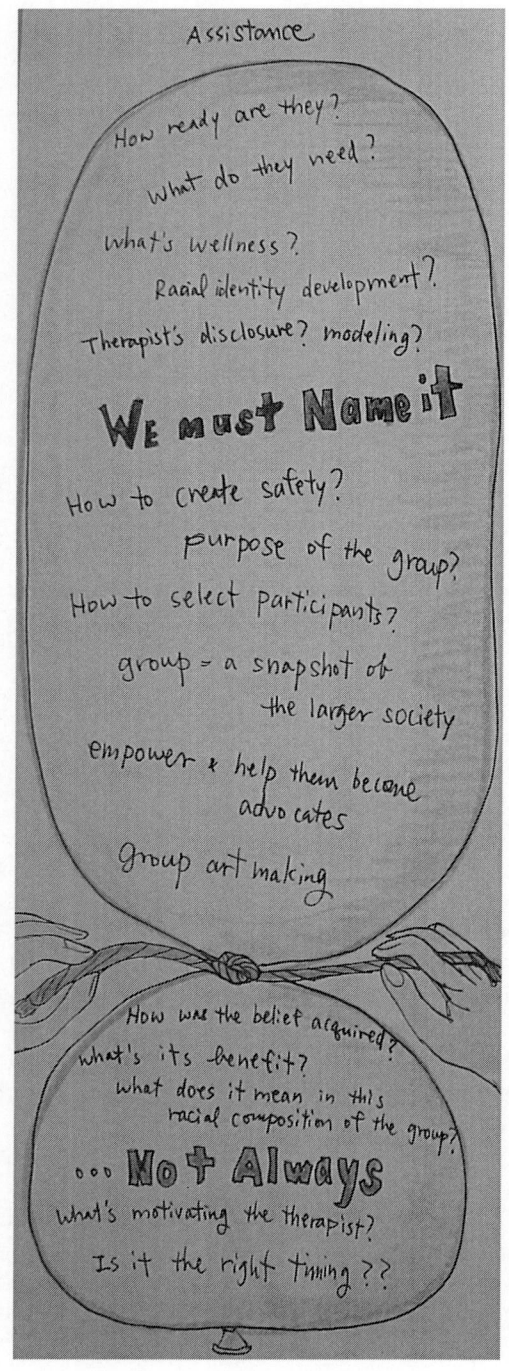

Figure 8.3 External assistance depicted as a balloon.

The two drawings for the assistance section show the process of sorting information, represented by a balloon. One drawing shows the external process of sorting assistance, categorizing it into two themes (i.e., "We must name it" and "Not Always") (see Figure 8.3). The bottom part of the balloon is much smaller, as more information supported the need for the art therapists to name Jane's racially charged comment in the group. In the second drawing, the bottom part of the balloon has been let go (see Figure 8.4). The remaining part of the balloon depicts the internal process of sorting assistance, determining how to execute the act of naming a racially charged comment in the group.

8.2.4 R-Responsibility/Risk

If Sarah and Kaori were to select Option One, they would fulfill their responsibility for Jane's well-being by protecting her from discomfort she may feel by having the racist nature of her comment discussed in front of others. On the other hand, this option increases the risk that other participants may feel neglected and maintain reduced trust with the art therapists, especially Sarah who discouraged discussing social justice; this may lead them to withdraw from subsequent sessions. Other participants may not feel they can relate to Jane, consequently affecting group cohesion.

If Kaori is to select Option Two, she first needs to discuss with Sarah her own discomfort related to how Sarah handled Jane's comment before they can start planning how to bring social justice issues back into the group work. Ratts et al. (2010) spell out some of the possible risks that arise when a therapist decides to include social justice in group work: "being vulnerable to attacks by colleagues; being seen as a troublemaker and outcast within the field; and stretching ethical limits and boundaries (p. 166)." Kaori would be exposed to these risks with Option Two, as there is a possibility that Sarah may see the group work differently and remain firm in her decision to not include social justice. If Sarah and Kaori decide to facilitate a discussion about race, they would fulfill their responsibility to group participants in that their feelings about Jane's comments (and possibly their experiences in the larger society) would be processed. However, Jane may withdraw from the group and Sarah may feel unfamiliar with and/or uncomfortable discussing social justice issues.

In the drawing exploring responsibility and risk (see Figure 8.5), Kaori is taking the lead to balance three balls on an umbrella. Whichever option Kaori and Sarah chooses, it is a given that they need to keep managing the group dynamic along the lines of the terms written on the balls: Jane's well-being, other participant's well-being, and group cohesion. Their ongoing responsibility to the group is symbolized with the metaphor of Kasa-mawashi ("Umbrella turning"), a traditional Japanese performance. One must continue turning the umbrella until the show stops in order to balance all the balls on top.

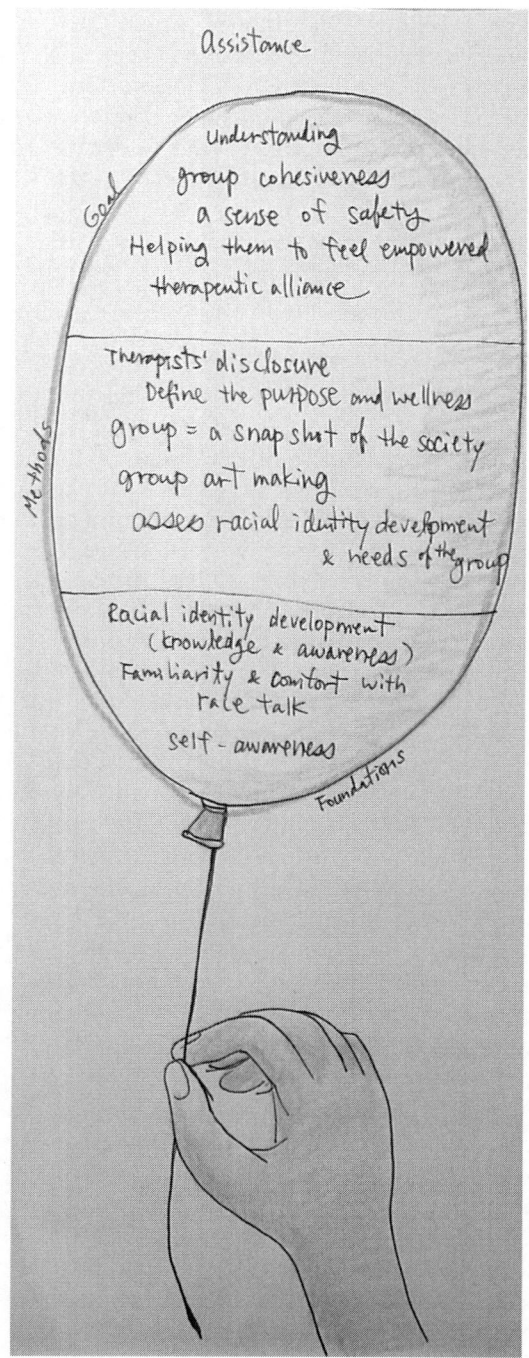

Figure 8.4 The lower part of the balloon was let go, and the remaining part
of the balloon shows how the writer organized recommendations.

8.2.5 T-Take Action

Overall, Option Two, which requires Kaori to facilitate a discussion about racism in the group alongside Sarah, seems to be the most ethical action. It is supported by American Art Therapy Association (2013) principle 1.1 to respect Jane's right and simultaneously facilitate Jane's understanding of the negative impact of her comments. American Art Therapy Association (2013) principles 7.1., 7.4., 7.5., and 7.7 hold the art therapists accountable for upholding the value of justice by discouraging discrimination, showing sensitivity to societal oppression, and striving for culturally sensitive interventions. In addition, American Art Therapy Association (2013) principle 10.5. calls for the art therapists to contribute to building a better community.

In Option Two Kaori and Sarah must agree on the purpose of the group and the definition of emotional wellness. They also need to decide who between them is going to lead group discussion. Based on the guidance given by consultants and literature, Kaori would suggest Sarah lead the discussion. However, if Sarah feels she lacks the skills to do so, Kaori may decide to start the discussion.

Kaori and Sarah can also suggest artmaking as a way to raise their consciousness. After acknowledging the racist nature of Jane's comment, the art therapists can ask group participants to describe their emotional reactions through art making (e.g., "Can you depict how you are feeling to be with others in the group right now?"). Another suggestion is for group participants to create images to describe beliefs about their own race (e.g., "Can you create an image of what it means for you to be Asian/Black/White/Latinx/Indigenous? How is wellness practiced in the racial or ethnic group that you identify with? What does it mean to bring that part of you to this group as we talk about wellness?").

It would be important for group participants to recognize that they are building the group culture together and that race is an element which influences this process. The group can cultivate understanding through group art-making such as an inclusivity mural. It may also be beneficial to suggest the ADDRESSING model by Hays (2008) as a guide for group participants to examine their intersectional identities including race and facilitate a discussion on what the group needs in order for each group participant to be able to show up with all of the identities they have. Drawing and collage materials can be made available, and group participants contribute their symbols/images to create a group mural that depicts the inclusive community they aspire to build. Each participant may have more than one symbol/image, as each person often holds multiple identities. After the mural is complete, group members can engage in discussions using the following prompts: What was your contribution in creating the mural? What was your role in the creative process? What is your role in making inclusivity happen in the group and

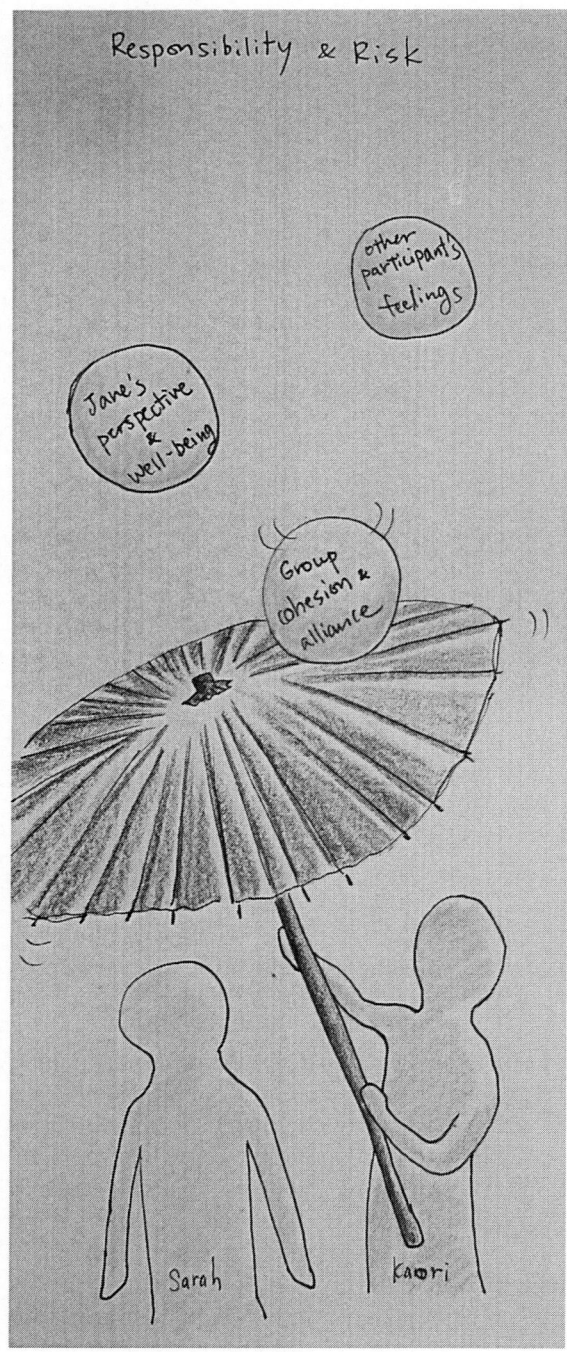

Figure 8.5 Group leaders juggling responsibilities.

in the larger society? How does your symbol relate to the rest of the mural? Is there any identity that was harder/easier to be incorporated? How did you collaborate or problem-solve with others in the group during the creative process?

In addition to discussing racism, another "-ism" visible in Jane's comment is ageism. Addressing her experience of ageism would also help Jane and other group participants understand how racism and other types of "-ism" affect one's emotional wellness. Sarah and Kaori can use Jane's previous art to start the conversation—what happens when the mandala has other people inside? What's the difference between her being alone in the mandala vs. having others around her? What emotions arise when she is surrounded by people of color, or who are younger? What does Jane think of the age of the figure being younger than her actual age? How do other group participants relate to her experience of being an older person?

In processing the action step, an image was created that depicts a scene of group art-making (see Figure 8.6). Both art therapists and group members are involved in the art making process, working on the same piece together. Speech bubbles illustrate that each person at the table has space to voice their thoughts. The image is framed in a circular shape, giving the impression of being contained despite the busy depiction of the group activity within the circle. While a circle was also a part of the image in the dilemma step (see Figure 8.1), the participants stood without any motion; In this step, the circle is bigger and embraces an engaged group of individuals within it.

8.3 Summary of the Main Concerns

When addressing social justice issues such as race in art therapy groups, art therapists need to consider their own racial identity development, participants' racial identity development, the group development phase, the group's needs, the group's readiness and capacity for discussing social justice issues, and the role participants play in the group relative to their experience in the larger society. Art therapists can use a variety of methods to facilitate social justice discussions, including self-disclosure, promoting group decision making, clarifying expectations and definitions, creating a sense of safety and respect among participants, connecting other "-ism"s to racism, and using structured activities or group art making. As group work is often a snapshot of the larger society, it is important for art therapists to strive to build a respectful, just, empowering, and inclusive culture in the group.

8.4 Tips for Avoiding Pitfalls

As the art therapy profession currently remains a Eurocentric and White dominant field, understanding of and proficiency with multicultural

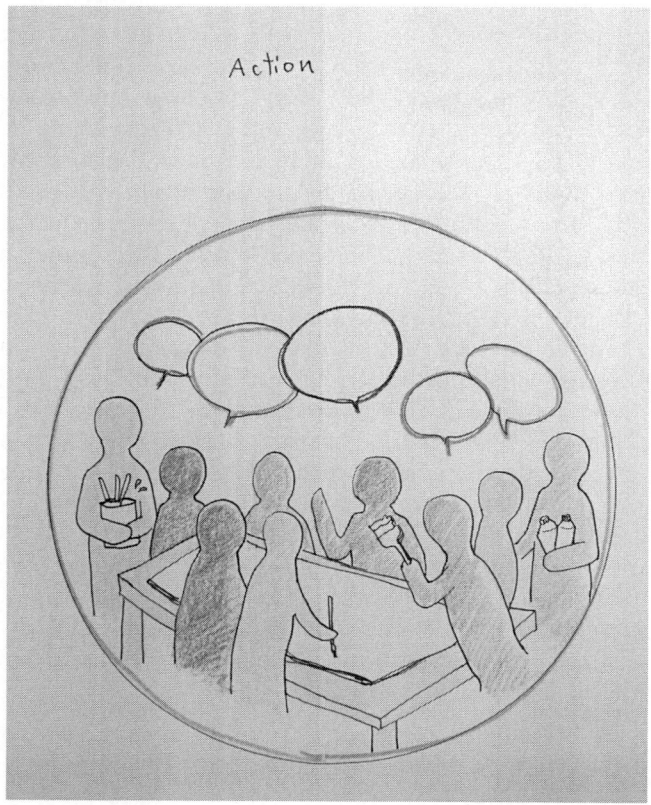

Figure 8.6 Group members and art therapists co-exist within the circle, as they do in the environment called the society. The image shows a lively discussion and group artmaking to imagine an inclusive culture together.

practice differs greatly among art therapists. When art therapists seek consultations related to multicultural practice, it is important to assess how much self-exploration a consultant or a supervisor has conducted, especially about their race, in addition to their knowledge of systemic oppression and privilege. In this regard, although studies suggest that therapists of color were more responsive to racial and cultural differences (Zaharopoulos & Chen, 2018) and tend to address race in therapy more than their White counterparts (Knox et al., 2003), art therapists of color should not be automatically assumed to be more knowledgeable to conduct social justice discussion than White art therapists. Those consultants who can provide wisdom are those who have processed their lived experiences through self-reflection on the meanings of their own race in the larger societal context.

When it comes to the handling of race and racism, art therapists may be well aware of the need to strive for culturally competent practice but find themselves unable to do so, due to barriers that exist outside of the ethical codes. These barriers are embedded in the societal, historical, and cultural contexts in this environment in which we practice art therapy. As important as it is to examine which ethical codes support or discourage discussions about racism and ageism in therapeutic settings, it is equally important to identify barriers that prevent well-trained art therapists from providing culturally competent care. Some barriers are: discouragement and lack of support from supervisors, colleagues, and agencies; the art therapist's implicit and explicit biases; lack of exposure to social justice discussions; intense emotionality related to the topic of race; and the art therapists' own racial trauma. As art therapists explore ethical ways to address social justice issues in therapy, it is imperative that they work to raise their own awareness of these barriers and identify ways to dismantle them.

8.5 Suggested Further Readings

Jackson, L. C. (2020). *Cultural humility in art therapy: Applications for practice, research, social justice, self-care, and pedagogy.* Jessica Kingsley.

Jackson, who is a board-certified art therapist and psychologist, describes cultural humility as a way to integrate social justice in art therapy. Each chapter in this book includes a reflective art exercise to raise the reader's awareness of their intersecting identities as well as how they inter-relate to others.

Menakem, R. (2017). *My grandmother's hands: racialized Trauma and the pathways to mending our hearts and bodies.* Central Recovery Press.

As a social worker who is trained in somatic experiencing therapy, Menakem guides therapists to understand the racial trauma and racial dynamics of the American society from the body-centered perspective. This book is helpful for art therapists to understand how their racialized bodies affect therapeutic relationships with clients.

Zaharopoulos, M., & Chen, E. C. (2018). Racial-Cultural Events in Group Therapy as Perceived by Group Therapists, *International Journal of Group Psychotherapy, 68(4)*, 629–653. https://doi.org/10.1080/002072 84.2018.1470899

This qualitative study explores racial-cultural interactions, processes, and incidents during group sessions. The authors interviewed group therapists to extract information on what type of racial-cultural events may impact group processes.

References

Alvarez, A. N., Liang, C. T. H., & Neville, H. A. (2016). Introduction. In A. N. Alvarez, C. T. H. Liang, & H. A. Neville (Eds.), *The cost of racism for people of color: Contextualizing experiences of discrimination* (pp. 3–8). American Psychological Association.

American Art Therapy Association. (2011). *Art therapy multicultural and diversity competencies.* https://arttherapy.org/wp-content/uploads/2017/06/Multicultural-Competencies.pdf

American Art Therapy Association. (2013). *Ethical principles for art therapists.* https://arttherapy.org/wp-content/uploads/2017/06/Ethical-Principles-for-Art-Therapists.pdf

Art Therapy Credential Board. (2021). *Code of ethics, conduct, and disciplinary procedures.* https://www.atcb.org/wp-content/uploads/2020/07/ATCB-Code-of-Ethics-Conduct-DisciplinaryProcedures.pdf

Bartoli, E., & Pyati, A. (2009). Addressing clients' racism and racial prejudice in individual psychotherapy: Therapeutic considerations. *Psychotherapy*, *46*(2), 145–157. 10.1037/a0016023

Burnes, T. R., & Ross, K. L. (2010). Applying social justice to oppression and marginalization in group process: Interventions and strategies for group counselors. *The Journal for Specialists in Group Work*, *35*(2), 169–176. 10.1080/01933921003706014

Corey, G. (2000). *Theory and practice of group counseling* (5th ed.). Wadsworth/Thomson Learning.

Hays, P. A. (2008). *Addressing cultural complexities in practice: Assessment, diagnosis, and therapy* (2nd ed.). American Psychological Association.

Helms, J. (2008). *A race is a nice thing to have: A guide to being a white person or understanding the white persons in your life* (2nd ed.). Microtraining Associates.

Jackson, L. C. (2020). *Cultural humility in art therapy: Applications for practice, research, social justice, self-care, and pedagogy.* Jessica Kingsley.

Kendi, I. X. (2019). *How to be an antiracist.* One World.

Knox, S., Burkard, A. W., Johnson, A. J., Suzuki, L. A., & Ponterotto, J. G. (2003). African American and European American therapists' experiences of addressing race in cross-racial psychotherapy dyads. *Journal of Counseling Psychology*, *50*(4), 466–481. 10.1037/0022-0167.50.4.466

MacLeod, B. (2013). Social justice at the microlevel: Working with clients' prejudices. *Journal of Multicultural Counseling and Development*, *41*(3), 169–184. 10.1002/j.2161-1912.2013.00035.x

Oulo, I. (2018). *So you want to talk about race.* Seal.

Potash, J. S. (2018). Relational social justice ethics for art therapists. *Art Therapy: Journal of the American Art Therapy Association*, *35*(4), 202–210. 10.1080/07421656.2018.1554019

Ratts, M. J., Anthony, L., & Santos, K. N. T. (2010). The dimensions of social justice model: Transforming traditional group work into a socially just framework. *Journal for Specialists in Group Work*, *35*(2), 160–168. 10.1080/01933921003705974

Sue, D. W. (2015). Race talk and facilitating difficult racial dialogues. *Counseling Today*. https://ct.counseling.org/2015/12/race-talk-and-facilitating-difficult-racial-dialogues/

Zaharopoulos, M., & Chen, E. C. (2018). Racial-cultural events in group therapy as perceived by group therapists. *International Journal of Group Psychotherapy*, *68*(4), 629–653. 10.1080/00207284.2018.1470899

9 Technology and Art Therapy: Navigating the Use of Digital Art and/or Telehealth in the Art Therapy Process

Faith Thayer

Rapid advancements in technology have had effects on multiple aspects of interpersonal relationships. These same technological developments have had significant ramifications on the therapeutic relationship in art therapy, giving rise to many new benefits while also presenting new challenges. Chief among these new challenges are novel ethical considerations and questions facing art therapists, both on the individual level and in the profession as a whole, ranging from changes in the nature of a clinician's privacy to questions about the quality of virtual care.

The utilization of novel technology and treatments in art therapy dates back to the Weinberg (1985) study of computer-aided art therapy treatment. A new development is a rapid increase in the accessibility of technological devices that make virtual methods for engagement widely available. For example, there has been an explosion of creative digital applications accompanied by a multitude of social media platforms that make it possible for creative content to be shared instantly (Choe & Carlton, 2019). Orr's (2012) survey found that while art therapists have adopted more technology into their practice, there have been reservations over ethical issues of incorporating technology (Orr, 2012). Over the past decade, there have been increased digital and online options for art therapists, including the ability to conduct sessions virtually, manage the scheduling and billing of sessions digitally, and advertise services online. Teletherapy increases options for where one can conduct the sessions, which devices to use, and the modality of how art is created, shared, and stored. Further, teletherapy expands communication options with patients, as well as provides flexibility for graduate-level art therapy training and continuing education. Each of these new options entails new and evolving ethical challenges.

There are both advantages and disadvantages to art therapists' use of telehealth and digital art-making in their practice. Zubala et al. (2021) reviewed the literature on technology in art therapy and concluded that there are both vast opportunities and severe risks. In a multi-database search yielding 249 publications, Stoll et al. (2020) found the most common ethical arguments in favor of online psychotherapy included the

DOI: 10.4324/9781003175124-9

expansion of access and availability, the financial advantages provided by technology that allowed for cost savings, and the increased methods available for communication between therapist and client. Some of the most common ethical arguments against online psychotherapy were questions about therapist competency stemming from a lack of training specific to the technology, issues of confidentiality in the digital world, and the relative lack of research into this growing field. In addition, art therapists may face numerous logistical challenges. For example, as highlighted in a survey by the American Art Therapy Association (2020), challenges may include the inability to view a client's art-making process and clients' lack of easy access to art materials in their own homes. As many facets of modern life are increasingly lived in the online digital space, it is reasonable to conclude that art therapists will face more questions than ever about the use and storage of digital imagery created in therapy.

9.1 The Case of Sara and Dorothy

Sara is an art therapist working in a private practice setting. To provide maximum flexibility for clients, she provides treatment via telehealth. Dorothy is an adult patient diagnosed with Anxiety and Autism Spectrum Disorder Level 1 (ASD). Dorothy had been in treatment with Sara for 8 months in weekly group and individual sessions, both in-person and via telehealth but is currently attending sessions exclusively via telehealth. The group treatment sessions are psycho-educational, focusing on social skills, and the main objectives for Dorothy's individual sessions focus on developing coping strategies for anxiety reduction and trauma-informed exploration of sensory-inducing triggers for meltdowns.

Using a HIPAA-compliant secure platform, the artwork is created in telehealth sessions using a shared whiteboard where both the patient and the therapist have control. Dorothy often utilizes photography in treatment by uploading photographs to a digital platform and then creating art pieces by drawing, cutting, and collaging the images virtually. During sessions Dorothy uses the chat feature, including the use of emojis, to convey her thought process. Dorothy will also often change her background image during sessions to photographs or artwork related to the content being processed with the therapist.

During a recent telehealth group session, one of the group members announced to the group that she saw a photograph of Sara on Dorothy's public social media page. In the group session, Dorothy stated that she forgot to crop that week's artwork screenshot before posting it to social media. Sara was surprised when Dorothy explained that she regularly posts images of the artwork created during her sessions as well as images of the sessions themselves. Dorothy stated that her posts sometimes include images of herself and Sara because these images, and backgrounds, complement the artwork. As Sara hears Dorothy talk about posting artwork from their sessions to social media, she feels unsure of how to proceed.

9.2 Analysis of the Case

In this situation, Sara could respond by creating a virtual gallery with Dorothy, which would bring her to the need to publicly share her in-session artwork into the therapeutic process (Option One). Alternatively, Sara could request Dorothy remove any in-session screenshots posted and request that she refrain from public exhibition of in-session artwork via social networks (Option Two).

9.2.1 D-Dilemma

9.2.1.1 Option One: Principles Supporting Option One

When consulting the American Art Therapy Association (AATA, 2013) *Ethical Principles for Art Therapists* and the Art Therapy Credentialing Board (ATCB, 2021) *Code of Ethics, Conduct, and Disciplinary Procedures*, there are multiple codes and principles to support Option One. By supporting Dorothy to create her exhibitions, Sara is obtaining the ability to support her in the process. She would be following American Art Therapy Association (2013) principle 5.8, where the therapist clearly defines where and when the exhibition will take place. She would then be able to work with Sara to make sure she clearly understands the ramifications of sharing work online with an audience, which would be in alignment with American Art Therapy Association (2013) principle 5.9, requiring the client to be aware of the widespread possibility of exposure when contributing artwork to an online exhibition. She would also be in compliance with American Art Therapy Association (2013) principle 5.5 that states the therapist must respect the client's choice to remain non-anonymous in the exhibition process.

American Art Therapy Association (2013) principle 15.3 states that the art therapist should discuss with the client the benefits and constrictions of teletherapy and assess whether the client has the cognitive ability to use electronic-assisted art therapy. Option One provides Sara with the opportunity to discuss electronic exhibition pros and cons with Dorothy and to assess Dorothy's comprehension of the process. Dorothy is diagnosed with ASD, and American Art Therapy Association (2013) principle 15.4 states that art therapists provide for communication that is accessible to persons with disabilities. Dorothy communicates verbally and does not have cognitive constraints, but Sara has experienced, via telehealth sessions, the significant way in which Dorothy is inclined to discuss highly emotional content within the chat function rather than verbally.

Dorothy has previously shared that she has found sanctuary in the non-verbal, sensory-friendly aspects of an online community. She also shared with Sara that she is an active member of neurodiversity social groups and that she identifies as an "Aspy," implying that she does not feel that her ASD is a disability. Further, American Art Therapy Association (2013) principle 4.0 states the art therapist regards artwork as the property of the client. Sara is honoring American Art Therapy Association (2013) principle 4.0 by providing Dorothy the images of the artwork to display.

9.2.1.2 Option One: Codes and Principles Discouraging Option One

There are American Art Therapy Association (2013) principles and ATCB (2021) codes that discourage option one. While the HIPPA compliant platform used for sessions is in accordance with current laws, regulations, and American Art Therapy Association (2013) principle 16.3, the same secure platform could not be used to facilitate an asynchronous art exhibition. Indeed, to use an appropriate platform would require using an invitation-only password-protected platform with encryption and downloading restrictions. This would limit the potential attendees and likely defeat the purpose of Dorothy having an online exhibition. Even with the above measures taken, Sara cannot prevent individuals from taking screenshots of the images. American Art Therapy Association (2013) principle 5.2 requires art therapists to ensure safe-guards when facilitating an exhibition, such as the client approving of exhibiting work. Although Dorothy may agree to have her work ex-hibited, she may not understand the full ramifications of who may end viewing the gallery. Once publicly posted, Sara may not be able to protect Dorothy from issues such as screenshot reuse or cyber-bullying. In short, even with the identified measures taken, limitations remain due to the nature of a virtual gallery. This also brings into consideration American Art Therapy Association (2013) principles 2.0 and 2.1, requiring that art therapists ensure confidentiality.

9.2.1.3 Option Two: Principles and Codes Supporting Option Two

If Sara were to request termination of the exhibition of Dorothy's art-work on social media platforms, she would be in compliance with American Art Therapy Association (2013) principle 15.0, which states the need for the therapist to take steps to ensure confidentiality when using social media platforms. Sara does not have the ability to control whether Dorothy continues to post artwork created during treatment on social media. This is in line with American Art Therapy Association (2013) principle 16.4 that requires the therapist to protect the client's identity.

American Art Therapy Association (2013) principles 1.3, 1.4, and 1.6 express the expectation of a clearly defined relationship between therapist and client: The art therapist must avoid introducing any ambiguity into the nature of the therapist-client relationship, both during and after treatment. Sara would clearly be in accordance with this by disapproving and insisting on the termination of any social network within the therapeutic process. Sara does not follow or "friend" any of her current or previous clients. Therefore, she cannot see the images Dorothy has posted. This is in line with ATCB (2021) code 2.3.1 that states that art therapists shall not engage in relationships outside of the therapeutic role, including relationships on social media.

9.2.1.4 Option Two: Principles Discouraging Option Two

American Art Therapy Association (2013) principle 1.1 directs art therapists to respect the rights of clients to make decisions and makes art therapists responsible for helping them to comprehend the ramifications of their decisions. If Sara pursues option two, one could question whether she is fully respecting Dorothy's decision to share her therapeutic process publicly.

If Dorothy does not comply with Sara's request to stop posting screenshots of sessions containing her images, then she could be forced to terminate therapy. Sudden termination of therapy could create a negative transition when Dorothy is already in a vulnerable state. This directly goes against American Art Therapy Association (2013) principle 14.6 that states an art therapist must be attentive to the possible negative reaction of the client to the termination.

In accordance with American Art Therapy Association (2013) principle 4.1, Sara had previously released artwork created during treatment to Dorothy to do with as she pleases. By informing Dorothy that she cannot do the same in virtual treatment, Sara is changing pre-established therapeutic norms, thereby setting conflicting therapeutic boundaries.

9.2.2 O-Outcomes

In this dilemma, the relevant parties are Dorothy, Sara, Sara's other patients including Dorothy's peers in group therapy, and Dorothy's online community. To process the Options and Outcomes step, Sara depicts an eyeglass showing her view of the possible outcomes for each option (see Figure 9.1). One eye is wide-open and alert, while the other is closed and at rest. The alert open eye depicts Sara's anxiety around the outcomes of Option One. The closed somber eye depicts outcomes of Option Two where Sara is at peace, but the artwork will not be seen by the greater virtual community.

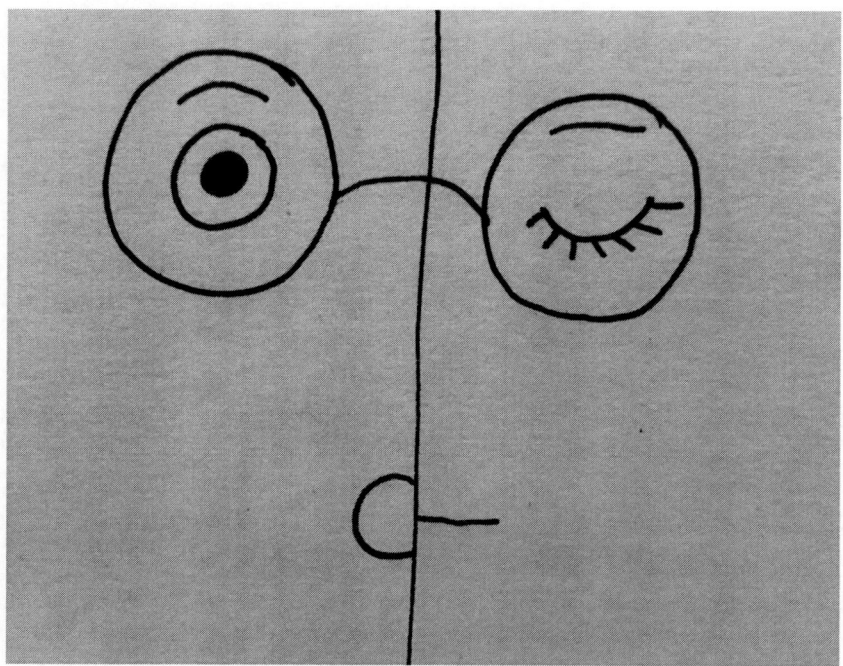

Figure 9.1 Options and outcomes.

9.2.2.1 Option One

If Sara creates a virtual exhibition on a separate, secure, non-social media website inaccessible to the general public, the exhibition will have a clear start and end date and be restricted by invitation. Sara can provide Dorothy a password and link to share with individuals in her community. There will be an exhibition flyer that Sara, if she chooses, can share in her social network, but interested parties would be required to apply for password access to the art gallery. Posting the artwork from the therapeutic sessions could provide support and validation for others in the virtual community going through the same process during a time of extreme isolation. The process of the exhibition could be an empowering experience and further Dorothy's sense of self and foster positive identity development.

It is also important for Sara to consider her responsibility to her other patients, especially the other members of Dorothy's group therapy, who may have emotional responses to Sara endorsing the exhibition process. Regardless of whether Sara offers the same option to other group members, there may be consequences given that an exhibition may or may not be in the best interest of each group member, in accordance with their individual treatment plans. By learning how to provide a virtual exhibition, Sara is potentially increasing her competence with telehealth practice skills and components. The publicity of an online exhibition may increase awareness of the field of art therapy. Finally, the greater clinical community could also perceive it as a form of advertisement for Sara's practice, which has its own implications.

9.2.2.2 Option Two

Dorothy may feel rejected or even stifled by Sara's refusal to endorse an exhibition process. Dorothy struggles with communication, in-dependence, and finding her voice in the world. Dorothy's habit of sharing her artwork online is evidence of an innate need to communicate socially. By imposing a restriction on Dorothy, Sara could inadvertently exacerbate negative feelings around previous communicative challenges and lack of control, which could negatively impact Dorothy's current treatment process. While Dorothy's greater online community and Sara's other patients would not gain the knowledge of Dorothy's art therapy process, this would not necessarily impact their current experiences.

9.2.3 A-Assistance

9.2.3.1 Assistance from Consultants

Sara sought assistance from her clinical supervisor and asked "Would it be in the best interest of the therapeutic relationship to set a clear boundary by insisting Dorothy remove the public digital art share, which contained an image of Sara, or face termination of treatment?" Sara's supervisor responded by stating that Sara is obligated to uphold the best practice of her license, and turning a blind eye to the posting of treatment session photographs on social media would not align with certain aspects of that defined obligation. The supervisor suggested the best practice would be to provide Dorothy her artwork images because clients have ownership over their artwork. The supervisor also pointed out that Sara does not have the ability to confirm Dorothy's compliance with her re-quest without befriending Dorothy on social media, which is not ethical. The supervisor advised Sara to start by thoroughly searching for online platforms that would pose the least risk of exposure to the client. The supervisor's response seemed to lend support in favor of creating a virtual exhibition.

Sara asked her therapy network (via colleagues in her peer supervision group) the following question: "With the increase of technology use among patients, have other art therapists experienced similar dilemmas?" She received a diverse set of answers. One colleague described a two-way encrypted text-based art therapy treatment modality she was using and campaigned for the need for art therapists to continue to embrace technology. Another colleague shared that she had used the web to advertise and sell a series of greeting cards that her patients designed in treatment as a fundraiser for their therapy clinic. She felt that the process was empowering to clients and brought mental health awareness to the community. These responses also seemed to lend support to the idea of creating an online exhibition.

To further process Assistance from Consultants, Sara created Figure 9.2 representing the process of obtaining diverse information from external sources. In the image, balloon symbols contain the data, and

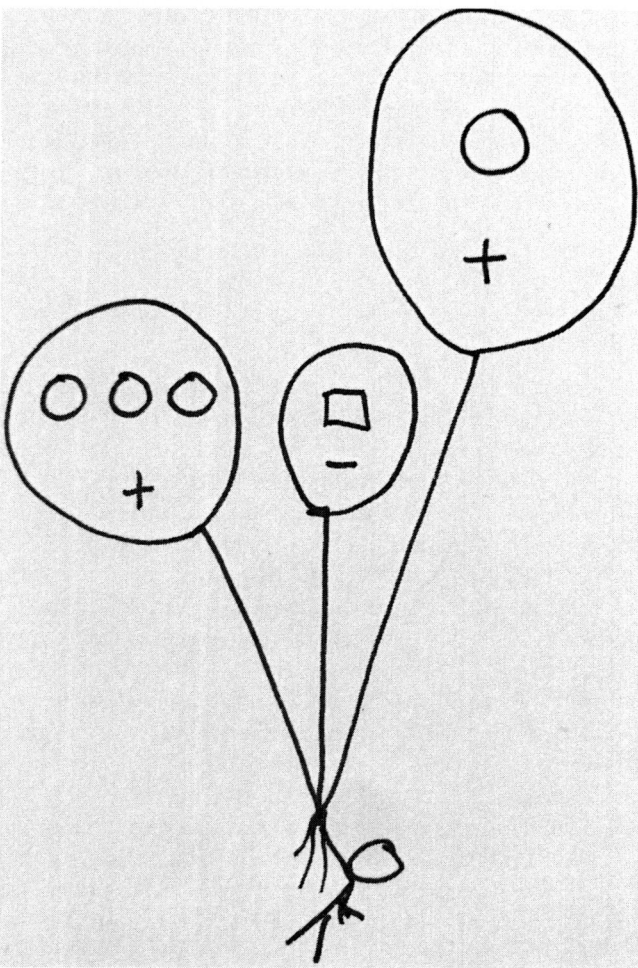

Figure 9.2 Assistance external.

Sara is floating from the strings attached to them, depicting the feeling of being lifted up from her state of conflict.

9.2.3.2 Assistance from the Literature

In *The Art Therapist's Guide to Social Media*, Miller (2017) describes the concept of digital social responsibility for art therapists. In deciding how to navigate digital spaces, art therapists need to consider four factors: (1) educational benefit, (2) maintaining privacy, (3) ensuring safety, and (4) having competence. Miller (2017) brings to light the concept of awareness and standards of digital boundaries for art therapists. Miller (2017) also identifies potential risks and benefits to clients sharing their artwork online. Risks may include vulnerability for criticism, the lack of restraint that can occur with online communication, the impact of unintended audiences having access, and the fact that once artwork is posted online it can never truly be permanently removed. Potential benefits are related to decreasing the stigma of mental illness, increased empowerment and autonomy, and increased socialization opportunities through social networks. Overall, Miller (2017) lends support to Option One, as Sara would educate herself further to uphold her digital social responsibility as an art therapist. Further, by creating a virtual gallery Sara would be opening up the opportunity for Dorothy to connect further with her virtual community.

The ability to find the support of a greater community in the virtual world is not just a possible benefit for clients but also for art therapists practicing in remote areas, as they have access to the support of other art therapists (Malchiodi, 2000). The ability of the art therapy community to overcome boundaries of distance, sensory, mobility, or safety by use of technology is not new. One example can be found in the work of art therapist Gudrun Jones in offering remote art therapy groups to cancer patients undergoing chemotherapy (BBC News, 2020). Other examples can be found in positive evidence findings for remote creative arts therapy studies supporting veterans' recovery (Levy et al., 2018; Lobban & Murphy, 2020; Spooner et al., 2019). Studies have found positive evidence supporting the need for technical support to overcome challenges set forth by a wide variety of atypical situations. These studies provide support for choosing Option One.

Carlton (2014) raised the possibility that art therapists might have a biased attitude toward technology use. In this case, Sara seemed to have a negative reaction towards having her image inadvertently taken and posted online without her knowledge or consent and it will be important to acknowledge that her negative reaction may bias her towards shutting down Dorothy's ability to share her artwork completely. Consequently, this source discourages choosing Option Two.

Alders et al. (2011) explored ethical challenges in technology-based art therapy, and stressed the need for repeated education and a hypothetical walk-through with clients who are posting artwork. Further, the art therapist has a responsibility to ensure clients have a comprehension of the repercussions of their online actions. Along the same lines, Choe and Carlton (2019) argue that American Art Therapy Association (2013) principle 5.2 is difficult to implement in relation to social media exhibition. These sources lend support for Option Two.

9.2.4 R-Responsibility/Risk

In this case, Sara faces potential risks from the relevant parties, which are: Dorothy, other patients including peers in group therapy, and her employer. These risks are depicted in an image where Sara is removing bricks from a platform that Dorothy is standing on, which represents the foundation of their therapeutic relationship. Sara is then repurposing the bricks into a wall, representing protection from client and clinician risk (see Figure 9.3). This image represents Sara's concerns surrounding her ability to consistently support the therapeutic relationship, while taking steps to prevent possible risk.

9.2.4.1 Option One

In choosing Option One, if the exhibition does not result in a positive development for Dorothy, or if her artwork is used in a manner she does not wish, she could file a complaint, or even a lawsuit, against Sara.

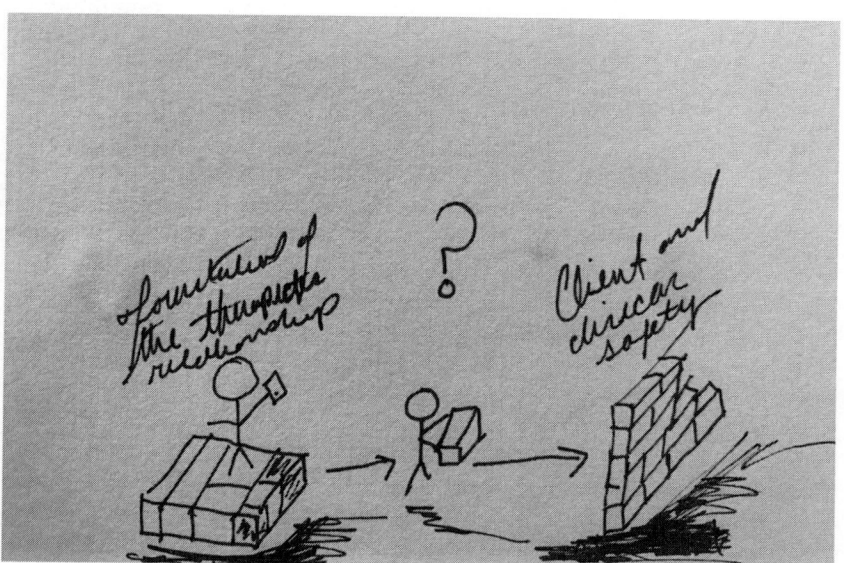

Figure 9.3 Responsibility and risk.

Further, Sara has a responsibility to her employer to provide therapy, and online artwork exhibition is typically not part of the therapy process.

9.2.4.2 Option Two

In pursuing Option Two, Sara is discouraging Dorothy's desired means of expression. By exercising her right not to be photographed and maintaining the ethical responsibility to uphold therapeutic boundaries, she may simultaneously be infringing on Dorothy's right to ownership of her artwork. If Dorothy terminates treatment as a result of not being able to share her work online, Sara may be liable for causing undue emotional harm as a result of the termination and not respecting Dorothy's digital culture.

9.2.5 T-Take Action

After considering both options, Sara concludes that Option One is the most ethical. Option One is supported by American Art Therapy Association (2013) principles 5.8, 5.9, 15.3, and 4.0. In addition, Option One creates a positive impact, protects the integrity of Sara's clinical practice, and furthers the therapeutic relationship between Sara and Dorothy. Option one also minimizes risks to Sara and is supported by the literature.

Sara creates an image representing the path that brought her to take action (see Figure 9.4). Depicted are uneven steps that transform from a ladder formation to a bridge-like image landing upon her final choice depicted as a computer. There are two pillars with eyes representing her assistance process. The windy steps represent Sara's process with obstacles and guidance that brought her to her informed final action of the virtual exhibition.

9.3 Summary of the Main Concerns

When incorporating digital art therapy into one's practice there are areas of ethical concern of which one needs to be aware. Due to the ever-changing venues and methods of telehealth-based art therapy, art therapists may find themselves working outside of their own competencies. This can manifest an abundance of ethical issues, such as breaches in appropriate data collection and storage. The level of privacy for not only the client but also for the clinician can be inadequate, resulting in the violation of confidentiality. Personal biases, including the ignorance of the continuously developing digital culture, can interfere with best practices. All the above concerns interfere directly with the required standard of care defined by the credentialing authorities.

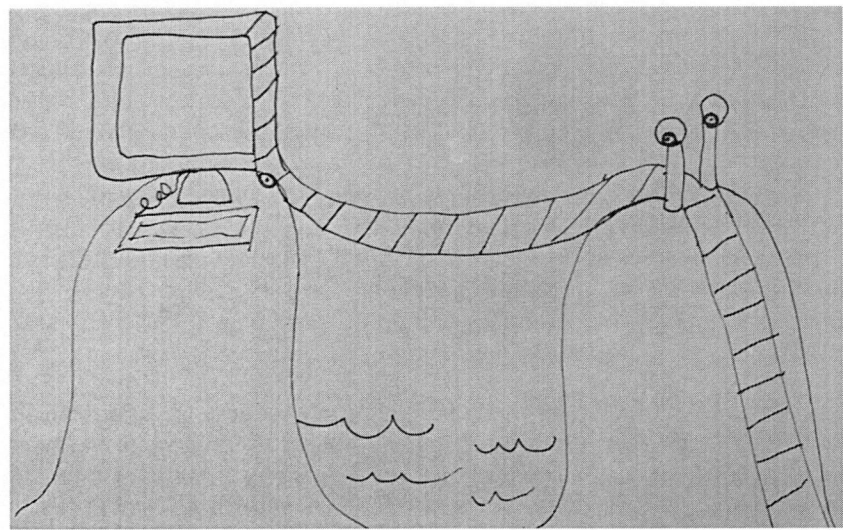

Figure 9.4 Take action.

9.4 Tips for Avoiding Pitfalls

The literature suggests that continuing education is necessary for the further integration of technology and art therapy (Belkofer & McNutt, 2011; Choe & Carlton, 2019; Miller, 2017). Education should include not only therapeutic methods and policy, but also a deeper exploration of all aspects of digital culture. Art therapists should actively seek out current research for supporting evidence-based digital art therapy practice.

Continuous reflection on clear boundaries and formal policies regarding virtual practice will help art therapists to be mindful of pitfalls, and clinicians should be cautious and deliberate in their own use of personal social media. As technology progresses rapidly, art therapy ethical standards, including informed consent policy, will need to be updated thoughtfully and continuously.

9.5 Suggested Further Readings

Choe, N. S., & Carlton, N. R. (2019). Behind the screens: Informed consent and digital literacy in art therapy. *Art Therapy, 36*(1), 15–21. https://doi.org/10.1080/07421656.2019.1565060

This article provides more information about possible concerns to art therapy providers, digital literacy skills, and recommendations for informed consent guidelines in electronic practice. Choe & Carlton discuss the importance of understanding digital media use in art therapy and how these techniques create both challenges and opportunities for art therapists. The importance of digital literacy among practitioners is underscored and guidance is given to developing an appropriate informed consent for digital media use with clients.

Miller, G. M. (2017). *The art therapist's guide to social media.* Routledge.

The book provides insights into the pros and cons of the use of social media in art therapy practice and its influences on the field.

References

Alders, A., Beck, L., Allen, P. B., & Mosinski, B. (2011). Technology in art therapy: Ethical challenges. *Art Therapy*, *28*(4), 165–170. 10.1080/07421656. 2011.622683

American Art Therapy Association. (2013). *Ethical principles for art therapists.* https://arttherapy.org/wp-content/uploads/2017/06/Ethical-Principles-for-Art-Therapists.pdf

American Art Therapy Association. (2020, August 14). *Art therapy during a mental health crisis: Coronavirus pandemic impact report.* https://arttherapy.org/blog-coronavirus-impact-report/

Art Therapy Credentials Board, Inc. (2021). *Code of ethics, conduct, and disciplinary procedures.* https://www.atcb.org/resource/pdf/ATCB-Code-of-Ethics-Conduct-DisciplinaryProcedures.pdf

BBC News. (2020, June 11). *Remote art therapy sessions for cancer patients.* https://www.bbc.com/news/uk-wales-53006595

Belkofer, C. M., & McNutt, J. V. (2011). Understanding social media culture and its ethical challenges for art therapists. *Art Therapy*, *28*(4), 159–164. 10.1080/07421656.2011.622684

Carlton, N. R. (2014). Digital culture and art therapy. *The Arts in Psychotherapy*, *41*(1), 41–45. https://doi.org/10.1016/j.aip.2013.11.006

Choe, N. S., & Carlton, N. R. (2019). Behind the screens: Informed consent and digital literacy in art therapy. *Art Therapy*, *36*(1), 15–21. 10.1080/07421656.2019. 1565060

Levy, C. E., Spooner, H., Lee, J. B., Sonke, J., Myers, K., & Snow, E. (2018). Telehealth-based creative arts therapy: Transforming mental health and rehabilitation care for rural veterans. *The Arts in Psychotherapy*, *57*, 20–26. 10. 1016/j.aip.2017.08.010

Lobban, J., & Murphy, D. (2020). Military museum collections and art therapy as mental health resources for veterans with PTSD. *International Journal of Art Therapy*, *25*(4), 172–182. 10.1080/17454832.2020.1845220

Malchiodi, C. A. (2000). *Art therapy and computer technology: A virtual studio of possibilities.* Jessica Kingsley.

Miller, G. M. (2017). *The art therapist's guide to social media.* Routledge.

Orr, P. (2012). Technology use in art therapy practice: 2004 and 2011 comparison. *The Arts in Psychotherapy*, *39*(4), 234–238. https://doi.org/10.1016/j.aip.2012.03.010

Spooner, H., Lee, J. B., Langston, D. G., Sonke, J., Myers, K. J., & Levy, C. E. (2019). Using distance technology to deliver the creative arts therapies to veterans: Case studies in art, dance/movement, and music therapy. *The Arts in Psychotherapy, 62*, 12–18. 10.1016/j.aip.2018.11.012

Stoll, J., Müller, J. A., & Trachsel, M. (2020). Ethical issues in online psychotherapy: A narrative review. *Frontiers in Psychiatry, 10*, Article 993. 10.3389/fpsyt.2019.00993

Weinberg, D. J. (1985). The potential of rehabilitative computer art therapy for the quadriplegic, cerebral vascular accident and brain trauma patient. *Art Therapy, 2*(2), 66–72. 10.1080/07421656.1985.10758788

Zubala, A., Kennell, N., & Hackett, S. (2021). Art therapy in the digital world: An integrative review of current practice and future directions. *Frontiers in Psychology, 12*, 1–18. 10.3389/fpsyg.2021.600070

10 Working with Vulnerable Populations

Melanie A. Peters and Jessica M. Hauck

As all mental health and medical professionals are aware, special care should be taken when working with vulnerable populations. Traditionally, this refers to children or minors, prisoners, pregnant women, mentally disabled persons, or economically or educationally disadvantaged persons. Recent literature also identifies other members of this population, including those with cognitive impairments or developmental delays, the elderly, those who are terminally or chronically ill, those with psychosis or severe/persistent mental illness, and others (Estrine et al., 2010; Han et al., 2018; Shi & Stevens, 2021). One specific area of concern identified was the increased risk of exploitation or coercion (Han et al., 2018), and the related need for caution when obtaining informed consent (Dobratz, 2004). Another identified issue was access to care (Shi & Stevens, 2021) and the need for alternative approaches (Estrine et al., 2010).

While a good deal of literature exists regarding vulnerable populations in general, evidence-based research specific to the field of art therapy is lacking. Interestingly, vulnerable populations are also not specifically mentioned in the *Ethical Principles for Art Therapists*(American Art Therapy Association [AATA], 2013). That being said, there are numerous informative case studies regarding the use of art therapy with terminally ill populations in hospice or palliative care. Common themes identified include using caution to avoid coercion, the need for compassionate and empathetic care, and utilizing alternative treatment approaches that may have a different purpose than traditional therapy (Burke, 2016; Collette et al., 2021; Dobratz, 2004; Han et al., 2018; Kim et al., 2008; Nainis, 2008; Rhondali et al., 2013; Youngwerth et al., 2019). The use of art therapy with this population has been shown to reduce anxiety, and depression (Collette et al., 2021; Youngwerth et al., 2019), while also reducing distress related to issues of change (Burke, 2016) and dysfunctional self-identity (Carr, 2014). Additionally, palliative care patients treated with art therapy have reported reduced pain (Collette et al., 2021; Nainis, 2008; Rhondali et al., 2013; Youngwerth et al., 2019), and improved visual perception and cognition (Kim et al., 2008).

DOI: 10.4324/9781003175124-10

The need for alternative treatment approaches in art therapy has been highlighted periodically in literature for several decades. One of the first influential pieces described the third-hand technique, first developed by Edith Kramer (Kramer, 1986, 2001). This technique can be thought of as a way of intervening therapeutically, and should be used to support or enhance a client's creative development, without being intrusive. It may be done verbally (e.g., cautioning a client that their hand may smudge the paper if they continue) or physically (e.g., holding a client's clay figure together while they reinforce it).

In recent years, art therapists have continued to build on this approach, further developing it for specific populations or issues; one of these newer models is the "Art on Behalf" approach (Ganzon et al., 2020), which was created to better support individuals with limitations related to their terminal illnesses, that prevented them from fully participating in traditional art therapy. Using this technique, the artwork is created by the art therapist, using only the patient's ideas and instructions (Ganzon et al., 2020). A growing body of research, many of which are also inspired by Kramer's 'third hand technique', investigate the impact of art therapists' direct involvement in treatment, including making art with clients during treatment (Teoli, 2020) or making response art (Franklin, 2010; Carr, 2014). Possible ethical concerns that have been identified include ownership of artwork (Ganzon et al., 2020), maintaining appropriate boundaries, and avoiding ambiguous relationships (Franklin, 2010; Teoli 2020). The issue of when to intervene or when not to intervene is also directly related to several aspirational principles for art therapists, including client autonomy (American Art Therapy Association, 2013).

10.1 The Case of Trevor

Trevor, a 25-year-old male, was referred to Katherine, an art therapist, after he began experiencing panic attacks and frequent angry outbursts upon being hospitalized and hearing his diagnosis of terminal cancer. As the only art therapist in the hospital system, Katherine explains art therapy services and Trevor agrees to enter into a therapeutic relationship with Katherine. The initial sessions are successful and Trevor actively engages in art-making. However, over the course of the next few months, Trevor's health declines and he enters into palliative care treatment. During the most recent art therapy session, Trevor states that he feels too tired and weak to physically make art. He shares with Katherine that he wants to continue to engage in art therapy services and asks Katherine if she would create the art for him while he verbally instructs her on what to do. Katherine is unsure of how to proceed.

10.2 Analysis of the Case

In the case of Trevor, the art therapist faces the ethical dilemma of deciding whether or not she should provide treatment where she allows her client to create the artwork by verbally instructing her on what to do. Given that Trevor meets the definition of a vulnerable client, special care must be taken to ensure treatment takes his unique circumstance into consideration.

10.2.1 D-Dilemma

Katherine's client, Trevor, is too weak to continue making art in sessions due to his terminal illness but suggests an arrangement where he will be able to continue with art therapy services, and creating art by providing instruction to his therapist. While both Katherine and Trevor believe that art therapy has been beneficial, Katherine is torn. On one hand, by agreeing to make the artwork she would be supporting Trevor's right to autonomy but this may alter the therapeutic relationship and create an ambiguity of roles. On the other hand, if she refuses to make the art she would remain within a typical scope of practice, but this may also cause harm to Trevor or the therapeutic relationship. In order to determine the most ethical course of action, Katherine consults the American Art Therapy Association's Ethical Principles for Art Therapists (2013) and analyzes the principles which may support or discourage each option. Katherine also engaged in art making and visually represented this step using a series of continuum lines (see Figure 10.1), with a dot representing the extent to which each principle supports the specified option; the paper was divided in half, with the left side representing the first option and the right side representing the second option.

10.2.1.1 Option One: Principles Supporting Option One

The first option is for Katherine to create the artwork in the session, as requested by Trevor, while she follows his instructions. This option is both supported and discouraged by a variety of ethical codes and principles.

By creating the artwork for Trevor, Katherine upholds American Art Therapy Association (2013) principle 1.1, which relates to client autonomy, and requires art therapists to respect the rights of clients to make their own decisions. Another principle that may support option one, is American Art Therapy Association (2013) principle 6.8, which insists that art therapists avoid engaging in behavior that may be demeaning. If Katherine refuses to create the artwork for the client, she may be invalidating his position as an expert of his own life. Collaboration with clients to create a plan for treatment is a vital part of the early stages of treatment. As such, American Art Therapy Association (2013) principle

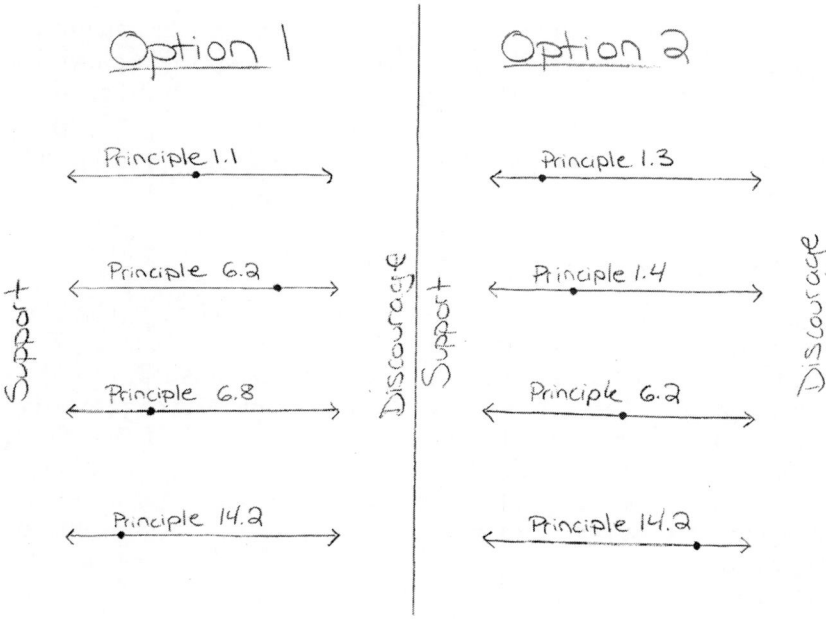

Figure 10.1 The dilemma stage is depicted with a series of continuum lines for
each ethical principle, with a dot representing the extent to which
each principle supports or discourages the specified option.

14.2 may also support this option since it encourages art therapists and
clients to work together to create treatment plans that will assist the client
in reaching their maximum level of functioning and quality of life. This is
especially relevant to the case since Trevor is a member of a vulnerable
population.

10.2.1.2 Option One: Principles Discouraging Option One

Although several principles support the option to create art for Trevor,
there are also several that discourage this option. Creating the artwork
for a client in session can be framed as a third-hand technique (Kramer,
2001). Katherine has limited experience with this technique, and as such,
this option would be discouraged by American Art Therapy Association
(2013) principle 6.2, which stipulates that art therapists must refrain from
using creative processes or therapy practices that are beyond their scope
of experience and training. Client autonomy is also relevant here. While
American Art Therapy Association (2013) principle 1.1 insists art
therapists respect the rights of clients to make decisions, it also requires
them to help their clients understand the consequences of these decisions.

Since Trevor's cancer is now terminal, it is likely that his ability to make artwork on his own will continue to diminish, a fact which he may not fully understand or be ready to process yet. This terminal illness also makes him part of a vulnerable population, which implies he is in need of additional protection from potential exploitation or coercion.

10.2.1.3 Option Two: Principles Supporting Option Two

If Katherine elects to not engage in this technique, inspired by a third-hand approach, she will need to find another acceptable treatment option for Trevor. As with option one, this second option is both supported and discouraged by a variety of ethical codes and principles.

By refusing to create the artwork for Trevor, Katherine may uphold American Art Therapy Association (2013) principle 6.2, by not using techniques that are beyond their scope of practice. This option is also supported by American Art Therapy Association (2013) principle 1.3, which directs art therapists to avoid ambiguity in the therapeutic relationship and maintain clarity about the different therapeutic roles that may exist. Choosing not to create the artwork could be one way that Katherine can avoid confusion about the therapeutic role. The act of creating artwork for clients, even if it's client-directed, is more typical in a non-therapeutic relationship. It is also inherently more personal. As such, this choice may also uphold American Art Therapy Association (2013) principle 1.4, which relates to avoiding multiple relationships.

10.2.1.4 Option Two: Principles Discouraging Option Two

Although several principles support the option to not create art for Trevor, there are also several that may discourage this option. American Art Therapy Association (2013) principle 6.2, which is related to experience and scope of practice, also suggests that art therapists provide referrals when the necessary treatment is beyond their scope of practice, but since Katherine is the only art therapist on this hospital unit, it is not possible to connect Trevor with an art therapist that is more versed in these types of techniques. Consequently, Katherine would not be able to uphold principle 6.2 and assist Trevor in obtaining other art therapy services. This option is also discouraged by American Art Therapy Association (2013) principle 14.2, which requires art therapists and clients to collaborate in designing treatment plans that support the client in maintaining the quality of life and the highest level of functioning. Trevor's condition is terminal, making it unlikely his level of functioning will improve, and his status as a member of a vulnerable population also creates a need for greater protection in this area.

10.2.2 O-Outcomes

In this case, the relevant parties who may be affected by either course of action are Trevor, Katherine, Katherine's other clients, her coworkers, and the art therapy profession as a whole. For each relevant party, Katherine must identify any foreseeable consequences if she were to take either course of action. To assist in this process, Katherine visually represented the weighing of her two options through the depiction of a scale (see Figure 10.2). On each side of the scale are words or images symbolizing any foreseeable consequences for each relevant party if Katherine were to proceed with either option.

10.2.2.1 Option One

By agreeing to make art for Trevor, Katherine would be using a flexible approach that is in line with Trevor's needs. This would benefit Trevor because it would allow him to continue to engage in services that could continue to enhance his quality of life. Trevor has also expressed that he finds therapy beneficial so Katherine may support his sense of autonomy especially since many aspects of Trevor's life are out of his control such as his terminal illness. However, Trevor may not fully understand that by

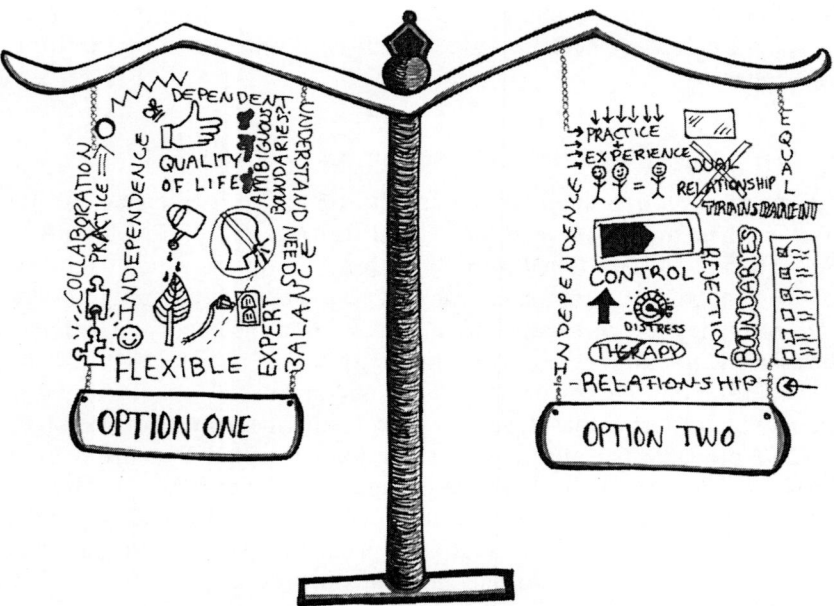

Figure 10.2 The options stage is represented by a scale weighing various words and images symbolizing any foreseeable consequences for each option.

instructing Katherine what art to create by proxy, he would no longer be physically creating the art which may damage his sense of independence and potentially lead him to feel like a burden. These impacts have the potential to create additional distress on top of Trevor's deteriorating physical state. In addition, if Katherine were to accidentally misinterpret Trevor's instructions or if the artwork doesn't come out how Trevor envisions, he may not feel comfortable letting Katherine know and may possibly feel as though Katherine does not understand him. This could further impact the therapeutic relationship.

Katherine's other clients could also be potentially impacted by this option. If her clients were to find out that she was making art for a client, they may feel as though Katherine is not providing equitable treatment. Further complicating this would be the fact that due to confidentiality Katherine would not be able to explain the circumstances of why she is making art in session for a client. This may damage her relationships with her other clients and potentially cause harm to the treatment process, or at worst cause her clients to discontinue services. To ensure that Katherine is practicing within her scope of experience, Katherine could further her competence in this area to ensure she is meeting Trevor's needs. This increase in the scope of competence might benefit future clients as she may be able to use this technique with clients in a similar situation as Trevor.

By being sensitive to her client's needs Katherine would be upholding the ethical principles of nonmaleficence and fidelity. This would benefit the art therapy profession because they would have professionals acting ethically and in the best interests of their clients. However, Katherine may also misrepresent what art therapy is to her coworkers by engaging in this option thus violating American Art Therapy Association (2013) principle 12.1 which states art therapists should represent themselves and the profession accurately. Her coworkers may assume that creating art for clients in session is something that all art therapists do. While this technique may be appropriate for this specific setting and population, it may not be appropriate elsewhere. However, by using art therapy in a nontraditional way in order to meet her client's needs Katherine may show how creative techniques can be successfully adapted to fit specific situations. This in turn would benefit the profession as a whole because it would positively contribute to the application of art therapy with vulnerable populations.

10.2.2.2 Option Two

Having a terminal illness, Trevor may be experiencing high levels of distress. By declining to make the art, Katherine may be taking away Trevor's means of self-expression and coping during this difficult time which may potentially cause harm and increased stress for Trevor.

Katherine may also invalidate Trevor's autonomy and expression of what he needs. Trevor may also feel rejected by Katherine's refusal thus hindering future attempts at collaboration in sessions. The therapeutic relationship may ultimately be negatively impacted because Trevor may feel as though Katherine is not listening or understanding what he needs. Consequently, Trevor may shut down and be uncomfortable being vulnerable with Katherine impacting the success of future sessions. At worst, Trevor may choose to discontinue therapy.

However, Katherine's refusal to make the art might also have the potential to benefit Trevor by compelling him to continue physically making art in sessions. Presuming he is able to do so, directly making art in session may boost his sense of independence and allow him to have more creative control over the finished products. Also, by setting clear boundaries and roles in the therapeutic relationship, Katherine minimizes Trevor's dependence on her. However, it should be noted that Trevor's physical state may continue to deteriorate to a point where he is unable to make any art in the future. Katherine could then help Trevor verbally work through the loss of his physical abilities, but this may not be beneficial to Trevor if he is strongly invested in art therapy treatment. Nonetheless, this option may benefit Trevor by protecting him from potentially being taken advantage of in his vulnerable state. Moreover, Katherine would not be perceived as using the situation for her own benefit in order to gain experience practicing a technique that is currently outside her scope of practice.

Katherine's other clients may benefit from this option because equal treatment would be occurring, thus upholding ethical principles related to fidelity and justice. By refusing to create the art for Trevor, Katherine herself may benefit by maintaining clear boundaries in treatment and avoiding a potentially ambiguous or multiple relationship with Trevor. The art therapy profession stands to benefit through the upholding of ethical principles related to maintaining boundaries and avoiding ambiguity (American Art Therapy Association, 2013). Indeed, option two protects the traditional therapeutic process of art therapy.

10.2.3 A-Assistance

To assist Katherine in the decision-making process, she should examine current literature, as well as consult with relevant professionals. The processing of information received in this step may be thought of in two phases, examining external information and processing it internally. The process of assistance was illustrated using a drawing of a large jar, with several smaller jars and vials being poured into it (see Figure 10.3). The different pieces of information gathered during this step are represented by the differently sized smaller jars, with main concerns written as labels. The swirls of ingredients in the large jar depict the weighing and consideration of different pieces of information.

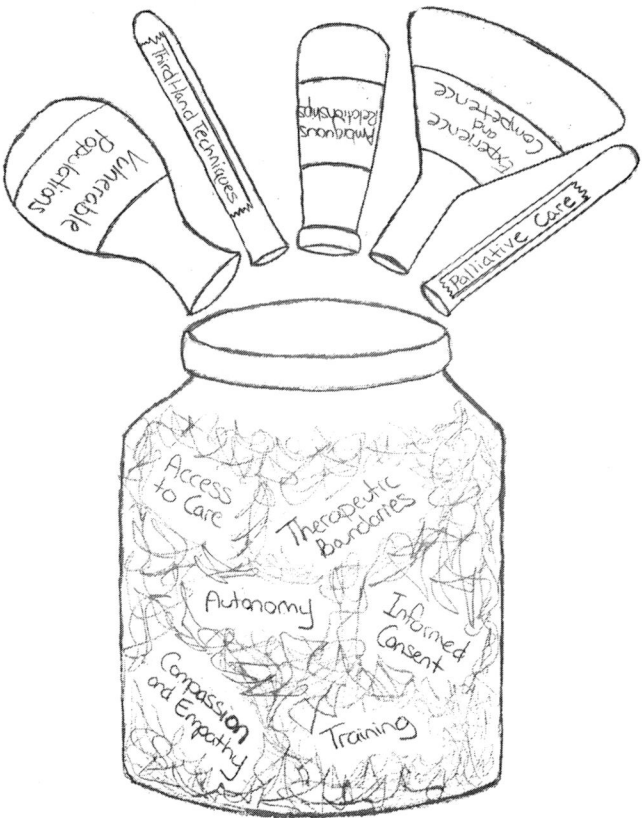

Figure 10.3 The weighing and considering of different pieces of information gathered from literature and consultation, represented by a series of smaller jars labeled with research topics, being poured into a larger jar with other ingredients.

10.2.3.1 Assistance from Consultants

The first area of the assistance step involves seeking consultation in alignment with American Art Therapy Association (2013) principle 1.7. This will help Katherine gain perspective to make a more informed decision. Katherine sought consultation on how to apply the ethical principles to vulnerable populations. Since vulnerable populations are not specifically mentioned in the Ethical Principles for Art Therapists (American Art Therapy Association, 2013), Katherine asked the ethics board if there are any additional concerns or responsibilities she should hold in this situation and inquired on whether this is seen as an ambiguous or exploitative relationship. The board representative indicated that this is a gray area, where caution should be used before proceeding. The board representative encouraged Katherine to seek legal counsel regarding local laws and regulations for working with vulnerable populations.

To gain clarification on the application of laws and regulations, Katherine consulted with an attorney familiar with mental health laws/regulations in the state/country where she practices and asked if she is violating any specific laws related to practice with vulnerable populations. The attorney indicated that while there were no laws that addressed this particular situation, she should nonetheless use caution to avoid potential exploitation of her patient.

10.2.3.2 Assistance from the Literature

The second area of this step involves seeking assistance from recent literature, to ensure current best practices are considered during the decision-making process. Specifically, research on the use of art therapy with vulnerable populations, and research examining the act of physically intervening, or artwork created by the art therapist. Evidence-based research on these subjects is limited, but numerous case studies have been useful and informative, beginning with landmark research regarding the use of Third-Hand techniques. This approach was described in detail by Kramer (2001), and was intended to be supportive without being overbearing. It involves the art therapist intervening verbally or physically in order to rescue from perceived failure or encourage success (Kramer, 2001). This piece of literature may lend support for the first option, making the artwork for the client, since Katherine would be protecting her patient from the sense of failure he may experience if he chooses not to make artwork himself or tries to and is unsuccessful.

Franklin (2010) discussed the act of creating artwork for clients, as a way of empathetically responding to the content of the session. This type of response art can be beneficial for some clients, but also comes with unique challenges. Specifically, art therapists must be aware of their own unconscious processes, and maintain effective and appropriate boundaries with the client in light of how this approach can feel overly intimate at times (Franklin, 2010). Even though Katherine would be making artwork as dictated to her by Trevor, this research seems to discourage the option for Katherine to create the artwork, since it may add ambiguity to the therapeutic relationship.

This boundary concern is also identified by Teoli (2020), in their discussion of the benefits of an art therapist engaging in art-making during group therapy. It was concluded that this process may benefit group members by increasing their engagement and improving the therapeutic relationship while making it more egalitarian (Teoli, 2020). However, ambiguous relationships in art therapy should be approached with caution, especially when working with vulnerable populations. Overall, this source seems to lend support for Katherine creating the art as it has the potential benefit of increased engagement.

The term vulnerable populations include minors, those with cognitive impairments or developmental delays, the elderly, those who are terminally or chronically ill, pregnant women, those who are economically disadvantaged, those with psychosis or severe/persistent mental illness, and others (Han et al., 2018; Shi & Stevens, 2021). Although the literature on vulnerable populations tends to encompass more than art therapy, the implications for the population itself still apply. As such, terminally ill individuals may be at increased risk for coercion or exploitation, and care should be taken when providing treatment. Dobratz (2004) indicated that when working with terminally ill populations, careful attention and assessment should also be used when obtaining informed consent, since this population may suffer from cognitive limitations related to their illness/treatment. Indeed, vulnerable populations may be easily coerced or in danger of exploitation (Han et al., 2018). One of the main issues this population seems to face is access to care (Shi & Stevens, 2021). The research on working with vulnerable populations using art therapy, seems mixed, with most indicating that caution should be used while simultaneously highlighting the need for compassionate and empathetic care, which may have a different purpose than traditional therapy (Burke, 2016; Collette et al., 2021; Dobratz, 2004; Han et al., 2018; Kim et al., 2008; Nainis, 2008; Rhondali et al., 2013; Youngwerth et al., 2019). Overall, this research seems to lend support for option one, allowing Katherine to support Trevor without denying him access to needed care.

Art therapy treatment in palliative care is a growing issue, which has received more research attention in past years, with an entire special issue dedicated to this topic in 2008 (Feen-Calligan, 2008). Art therapy with palliative care patients seems to have a positive impact in terms of reducing pain (Collette et al., 2021; Nainis, 2008; Rhondali et al., 2013; Youngwerth et al., 2019), anxiety, and depression (Collette et al., 2021; Youngwerth et al., 2019), while also reducing distress and confronting issues of change (Burke, 2016), and even improving visual perception and cognition (Kim et al., 2008). Overall, this combined palliative/hospice research seems to support the option to create the artwork, while also identifying several concerns. As with vulnerable populations in general, access to care is also an issue for palliative care patients, and Katherine is aware that she has limited referral options for Trevor. However, if she chooses to create the art, she also needs to assess Trevor's cognitive functioning before obtaining informed consent, to ensure no coercion is taking place while also making sure he understands the nature of their therapeutic relationship.

Ganzon et al. (2020) described a series of case studies on patients in palliative care who were treated with an "Art on Behalf" approach and highlighted the potential benefits and pitfalls of creating art on behalf of clients. This approach was created to better support individuals with limitations that prevent them from fully participating in traditional art therapy. In this model, the artwork is created by the art therapist, using only the patient's ideas and instructions (Ganzon et al., 2020); it is inspired by Edith Kramer's Third-Hand approach, but with notable differences, specifically regarding who actually creates the artwork (Kramer, 2001). Indeed, potential issues identified in this case study include the ownership of artwork created in session; the authors indicated that the artwork belongs solely to the patient. These case studies described numerous benefits, including meaningful communication, tangible evidence of their experience, and further engagement in artmaking (Ganzon et al., 2020). Although the authors acknowledge that their research is based on their interpretation, and not on the reported experiences of patients and their families (Ganzon et al., 2020), overall, this case series seems to lend support for the option of Katherine creating the artwork on behalf of Trevor, at his instruction.

10.2.4 R-Responsibility/Risk

Katherine must identify the relevant parties to whom she has a responsibility, as well as consider strategies for limiting liability before deciding which course of action to take. In this case, Katherine faces potential risks from Trevor, her other clients, her coworkers, and the art therapy profession. For this step, Katherine represents the management of her responsibilities through the Draw-a-Person-in-the-Rain assessment (see Figure 10.4). There is heavy rain with storm clouds above; however, the sun is peeking out from behind the clouds representing Katherine's various responsibilities to Trevor being fulfilled if she were to choose option one. There are puddles on the ground representing some higher-risk scenarios that Katherine would need to navigate with extra caution and further consideration. Finally, the person is holding an umbrella that is just large enough to protect them from the rain showing that while there are various risks involved in this option, there are many things Katherine could do to mitigate these risks.

10.2.4.1 Option One

By meeting Trevor where he is at and respecting Trevor's assessment of his needs Katherine would be fulfilling her responsibility to Trevor as her client because she would be fostering autonomy and respecting his position as the expert of his own life. Katherine would also be acting in the best interest of her client which would fulfill her responsibility to the art therapy profession as well as Trevor thus limiting risk. However, if Katherine decides to make the art with Trevor's instruction she may be ethically at risk for practicing outside her scope of practice. If Katherine

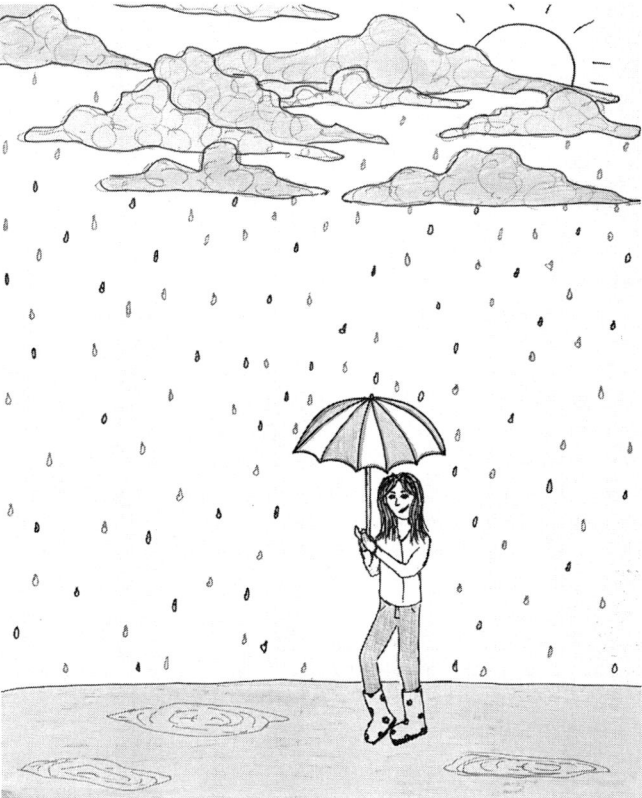

Figure 10.4 The responsibility/risk stage is depicted using a version of the Draw-a-Person-in-the-Rain assessment with each component representing the various risks involved in choosing option one as well as possible protective factors.

uses this technique she could also be at an increased risk of being sued by Trevor if it is not beneficial or if it is used incorrectly causing more harm to Trevor. Katherine could limit liability and also fulfill her responsibility to Trevor in this instance by first discussing any potential consequences of this choice with Trevor. She would also need to discuss how their relationship may be impacted as well as disclose her limited experience in creating art for clients in session.

To further limit liability, Katherine may choose to revise her informed consent and have Trevor resign to signify his understanding of what was discussed. Choosing this option may also come with an increased risk from her other clients. If Katherine's other clients at the hospital find out they are not being provided equal services or that they are not being given the same options for services as Trevor they could potentially seek legal action. To limit liability Katherine could offer the same option of making art in sessions with instruction to her other clients to ensure equity; however, this may cause further ethical dilemmas that would need to be considered by Katherine.

10.2.4.2 Option Two

By choosing to not make the art, Katherine limits the risk to herself and her coworkers because she would not be using a technique that she has no experience applying therapeutically. This also serves to limit liability and decrease the chance of legal action being taken against herself or Trevor's treatment team (Katherine's coworkers), for using a technique incorrectly and/or causing harm to Trevor. Even if Katherine discusses the potential consequences of making art with his instruction, Trevor may not fully grasp the impact this may have on him or the therapeutic relationship in the future. So, by not making the art Katherine could protect her client from making a decision that he may not fully understand the consequences of. By setting clear boundaries Katherine would also protect the therapeutic process as well as keep the therapeutic relationship strictly professional. This may protect Katherine from any unethical ambiguity in her relationship with Trevor thus limiting risk in this area. Katherine would also be limiting risk from her other clients because she would be treating all clients equally.

While Katherine may decrease liability by not making art for Trevor she may also increase risk by denying services to someone who is terminally ill as well as vulnerable and who cannot get services elsewhere at this time due to being hospitalized. By refusing to help Trevor, Trevor's mental and emotional states may deteriorate potentially causing harm to Trevor. Trevor in this instance could sue Katherine, his treatment team, or the hospital itself for being refused services and for not being provided the help he needs. Katherine could attempt to limit risk in this situation by discussing with Trevor her reasons for refusing to make the art for him as well as any foreseeable consequences of doing so. She may also discuss how therapeutic services can continue to be beneficial to Trevor without her making art for him during their sessions and potential alternatives to making art that fall within her scope of practice such as art viewing.

10.2.5 T-Take Action

After analyzing the case of Trevor, the most ethical option seems to be the first option, which involves Katherine making the artwork for Trevor in session, as requested. This option is supported by American Art Therapy Association (2013) principles 1.1, 6.2, 6.8, and 14.2. While principles 1.1 and 6.2 may also discourage this option depending on how they are interpreted, there is more evidence to suggest they support the option to create the artwork, since by choosing this option Katherine would be respecting the rights of clients to make decisions and would not be leaving her patient without the support given that she has no options for the referral. Several other American Art Therapy Association (2013) principles also discourage this option, including 1.3 and 1.4, but these relate to ambiguity in relationships and multiple relationships, and are outweighed because Katherine will be taking steps to explain the impact this may have on their relationship. In addition, the first option would benefit Trevor, who would get the opportunity to use art therapy services in a manner that works for him. This option would also benefit Katherine and her future clients, since it would help her gain experience and competence in this area, broadening her scope of practice.

This first option is also supported by recent literature, highlighting the potential value of creating artwork on behalf of clients, when they are unable to do so themselves (Ganzon et al., 2020). When working with vulnerable populations, including those like Trevor, there is an increased need to use caution to avoid potential exploitation. In choosing the first option, Katherine will be making Trevor's artwork for him, at his instruction, and solely for his benefit. Once she obtains an updated informed consent, attempting to provide more clarification on her therapeutic role and the relationship, this will further minimize her risk. This option also minimizes risk by ensuring Katherine fulfills her responsibility to Trevor, by providing art therapy treatment in accordance with the art therapy values of autonomy, beneficence, justice, and creativity.

In order to process this decision, Katherine chose to use the Bridge Drawing to show her overall process of coming to the conclusion of making art for Trevor with his verbal instruction (see Figure 10.5). The image shows a large pile of rocks and an unclear path leading up to the bridge symbolizing Katherine's initial reaction of uncertainty and not knowing which option to choose. The first section of the bridge is unstable with no support and missing pieces. This symbolizes Katherine not having enough information to make a decision and the possible missteps she could make along the way especially early on in the decision-making process. As the bridge continues, missing pieces are filled in as Katherine gathers more information and supports are added showing the various forms of assistance she received along the way. Once Katherine makes it to land on the right side of the page there is a clear path with a clear choice to make. Katherine depicted herself as ¾ of the way across the bridge because she still has many steps to take, such as discussing consequences and limitations with Trevor as well as creating a new informed consent, before implementing this course of action fully.

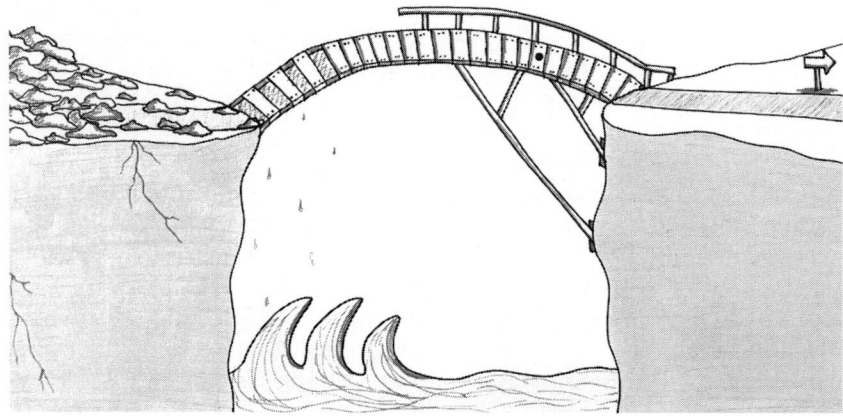

Figure 10.5 The take action stage is depicted through the use of a bridge showing the various steps the art therapist needed to make during the decision-making process to reach which course of action to take.

10.3 Summary of the Main Concerns

While much of the literature regarding vulnerable populations are focused on their involvement in research, a great deal of art therapy research exists regarding art therapy treatment for those with terminal illnesses. Although this can be a difficult population to work with, and there is still a need for more evidence-based research on these populations, art therapy seems to fill a need in the palliative treatment of terminal illness. Those with terminal illnesses, and vulnerable populations in general, may be susceptible to coercion or exploitation, especially when it comes to informed consent. When working with terminally ill patients, art therapists must use caution to be sure they are practicing ethically, in light of these additional considerations.

Another concern with this population, and with the use of 'third hand' inspired techniques, is ownership of the artwork. If the art therapist makes art for the patient in sessions, even with their verbal instruction, it might be unclear to whom the artwork belongs once complete. Traditionally, the person who creates the artwork owns the artwork, but this art-making process is more collaborative. However, Ganzon et al. (2020) identified that when making art on behalf of clients, the identified patient should be the sole owner of the artwork. This should be fully explained to the patient during the informed consent process, and repeatedly throughout care. This means that the art also remains part of the patient's record, and if they are ever discharged from care, they should have the option to take it with them.

A final concern with vulnerable populations, specifically those with a terminal illness, is the impact of their physical health and related sensory needs and sensitivity, and potential immunocompromised status. This increases the importance of using odorless materials, and fully disinfecting between patients. Also related to this, is the often degenerative nature of the terminal illness. Patients may choose to not make their own art due to not wanting to use what little energy they have left to engage in artmaking. That being said, as their condition deteriorates, there is also a risk that if they change their mind later in treatment, and want to create the artwork but are physically unable to do so, this could be damaging to the therapeutic relationship. While it has been found that there are many benefits to art therapists creating artwork in session for their terminally ill clients (Ganzon et al., 2020), there are also benefits to clients making their own art that the patient may no longer receive if they don't physically engage in art-making. Therefore, prior to agreeing to make the art, the art therapist should consider how hard to push them to continue creating their own art while they are still able to do so.

10.4 Tips for Avoiding Pitfalls

Vulnerable populations may be susceptible to coercion or exploitation. As such, caution should be taken when obtaining informed consent, specifically regarding the therapeutic relationship. Since terminal illnesses may have a cognitive impact, it is important that this be an ongoing process. In addition, when using third-hand techniques, ownership of artwork may become unclear. Research suggests that the identified patient should be the sole owner of the artwork, and the artwork (or images of the artwork) should be considered part of the client's record. Due to the nature of the terminal illness, art therapists should also be prepared to work closely with their patient's family members, who may be involved in care. Art therapists may also want to consider discussing ownership of the artwork with clients and their families, to determine who it will belong to once the patient is deceased, even if they've been discharged from care. Since terminal illness is often somewhat degenerative, physically, prior to agreeing to make the art, the art therapist should consider how hard to push them to continue creating their own art while they are still able to. Lastly, due to possible sensory needs and immunocompromised status, art therapists should be careful to use odorless materials, and fully disinfect all supplies between patients.

10.5 Suggested Further Readings

Ganzon, C., O'Callaghan, C., Dwyer, J. (2020). "Art on Behalf": Introducing an accessible art therapy approach used in palliative care. *The Arts in Psychotherapy, 67*, 101616. https://doi.org/10.1016/j.aip.2019.101616
    This series of case studies describe art therapy treatment in palliative care, using an "Art on Behalf" approach, where art therapists created art for patients, based on their conceptualization. Ganzon et al. (2020) identified potential therapeutic benefits of art therapy treatment using

this approach, including: meaningful communication, tangible evidence of their experience, and further engagement in artmaking. The authors also identify barriers that prevent this population from engaging in traditional art therapy as well as potential concerns of using this alternative approach such as ownership of the artwork.

Collette, N., Güell, E., Fariñas, O., & Pascual, A. (2020). Art Therapy in a Palliative Care Unit: Symptom Relief and Perceived Helpfulness in Patients and Their Relatives. *Journal of Pain and Symptom Management, 61*(1), 103–111. https://doi.org/10.1016/j.jpainsymman.2020.07.027

This clinical study investigates the potential benefits of art therapy in palliative treatment, including its impact on symptomatology. Collette et al. (2021) designed a pre-post single-arm intervention study, which also included the descriptive study of benefits, to further evaluate the outcomes of advanced cancer patients treated with art therapy interventions. The authors used evidenced-based assessment to collect data regarding experiences of pain, anxiety, depression, and well-being.

Nainis, N. A. (2008). Approaches to art therapy for cancer inpatients: Research and practice considerations. *Art Therapy, 25*(3), 115–121. https://doi.org/10.1080/07421656.2008.10129597

In this article, Nainis (2008) reflects on the unique needs of palliative care patients receiving art therapy treatment, while also discussing barriers to treatment and patient refusal of receiving treatment. The author also describes her experiences providing interventions in a pilot study, where art therapy was demonstrated to provide statistically significant reductions in cancer symptoms. Specific concerns included those related to sensory needs, physical abilities, limited time/energy, weakened immune systems, and other health concerns.

Shi, L., & Stevens, G. D. (2021). *Vulnerable populations in the United States* (3rd ed.). John Wiley & Sons.

In this nonfiction book, researchers Shi and Stevens (2021) draw on their experience in public health to provide a framework for working with vulnerable populations. Although this text is not specific to art therapy treatment or palliative care, it provides a wealth of information on specific concerns and considerations faced by vulnerable populations. The authors provide detailed, and up-to-date data on current trends in terms of disparities of care, and include relevant examples. This latest edition covered recent policy changes and their impacts on the accessibility of care.

References

American Art Therapy Association. (2013). *Ethical principles for art therapists.* https://arttherapy.org/wp-content/uploads/2017/06/Ethical-Principles-for-Art-Therapists.pdf

Burke, A. (2016). Catheters & canvases-using art therapy in palliative care. *Kai Tiaki: Nursing New Zealand, 22*(11), 28. https://search.proquest.com/docview/1902028292/fulltextPDF/9C1AEADA15F6485APQ/1?accountid=26523

Carr, S. M. (2014). Revisioning self-identity: The role of portraits, neuroscience and the art therapist's 'third hand'. *International Journal of Art Therapy, 19*(2), 54–70. 10.1080/17454832.2014.906476

Collette, N., Güell, E., Fariñas, O., & Pascual, A. (2021). Art therapy in a palliative care unit: Symptom relief and perceived helpfulness in patients and their relatives. *Journal of Pain and Symptom Management, 61*(1), 103–111. 10.1016/j.jpainsymman.2020.07.027

Dobratz, M. C. (2004). Issues and dilemmas in conducting research with vulnerable home hospice participants. *Journal of Nursing Scholarship, 35*(4), 371–376. 10.1111/j.1547-5069.2003.00371.x

Estrine, S. A., Hettenbach, R. T., Arthur, H., & Messina, M. (Eds.). (2010). *Service delivery for vulnerable populations: New directions in behavioral health.* Springer Publishing Company.

Feen-Calligan, H. (Ed.). (2008). Special issue on art therapy in palliative care [Special issue]. *Art Therapy, 25*(3), 1–146.

Franklin, M. (2010). Affect regulation, mirror neurons, and the third hand: Formulating mindful empathic art interventions. *Art Therapy, 27*(4), 160–167. 10.1080/07421656.2010.10129385

Ganzon, C., O'Callaghan, C., & Dwyer, J. (2020). "Art on Behalf": Introducing an accessible art therapy approach used in palliative care. *The Arts in Psychotherapy, 67*, 101616. 10.1016/j.aip.2019.101616

Han, C. J., Chi, N. C., Han, S., Demiris, G., Parker-Oliver, D., Washington, K., Clayton, M. F., Reblin, M., & Ellington, L. (2018). Communicating caregivers' challenges with cancer pain management: An analysis of home hospice visits. *Journal of Pain and Symptom Management, 55*(5), 1296–1303. 10.1016/j.jpainsymman.2018.01.004

Kim, S. H., Kim, M. Y., Lee, J. H., & Chun, S. I. (2008). Art therapy outcomes in the rehabilitation treatment of a stroke patient: A case report. *Art Therapy, 25*(3), 129–133. 10.1080/07421656.2008.10129593

Kramer, E. (1986). The art therapist's third hand: Reflections on art, art therapy, and society at large. *American Journal of Art Therapy. 24*(3), 71–86.

Kramer, E. (2001). *Art as therapy: Collected papers.* L. A. Gerity (Ed.). Jessica Kingsley Publishers.

Nainis, N. A. (2008). Approaches to art therapy for cancer inpatients: Research and practice considerations. *Art Therapy, 25*(3), 115–121. 10.1080/07421656.2008.10129597

Rhondali, W., Lasserre, E., & Filbet, M. (2013). Art therapy among palliative care inpatients with advanced cancer. *Palliative Medicine, 27*(6), 571–572. 10.1177/0269216312471413

Shi, L., & Stevens, G. D. (2021). *Vulnerable populations in the United States* (3rd ed.). John Wiley & Sons.

Teoli, L. A. (2020). Art therapists' perceptions of what happens when they create art alongside their clients in the practice of group therapy. *The Arts in Psychotherapy, 68*, 101645. 10.1016/j.aip.2020.101645

Youngwerth, J., Kutner, J., Somes, L., Jones, A., & Wibben, A. (2019). Integrating creative art therapy with palliative care (QI743). *Journal of Pain and Symptom Management, 57*(2), 479–480. 10.1016/j.jpainsymman.2018.12.252

11 Supervision and Professional Training

Jill McNutt and Erin Hein

The relationship between a supervisor and a supervisee is an important one to the education of new art therapists. A supervisor fulfills many roles within a supervision relationship (Barnett & Molzon, 2014). These roles include being an instructor and mentor, molder of the supervisee's professional development, encouraging self-exploration, and evaluating the supervisee (Barnett & Molzon, 2014). These roles ensure that supervisees are able to learn and ultimately are ready to embark into the field as a professional. With so much at stake in this relationship, ethical risks can easily sneak up on a supervisor. For example, supervision carries the possibility of dual relationships (Carrigan, 1993; Kurpius & Gibson, 1991). A supervisor is often looked upon to not only instruct a student but also teach the supervisee how to work through transference and counter-transference issues; this can often require self-disclosure and therefore resemble a therapeutic encounter. The supervision relationship can also result in an imbalance of power between the involved parties (Kurpius & Gibson, 1991; Ellis et al., 2014). Since supervisors are evaluators of supervisee progress; a supervisee may, consciously or unconsciously, behave a specific way or withhold concerns in order to receive a favorable evaluation. Supervisees may interact with clients in a therapeutic manner with theoretical knowledge and no past experience; therefore, there is a lot of responsibility on supervisors to maintain the quality of the education and correct issues early (Barnett & Molzon, 2014).

To ensure a supervisor has the information needed to best work with a supervisee, the American Art Therapy Association (American Art Therapy Association, 2013) and Art Therapy Credentialing Board (ATCB, 2021) have sections in their codes of ethics and principles addressing the supervisory relationship. These guide how to responsibly supervise, how to prevent ethical issues, as well as address them when they arise.

11.1 The Case of Jane and Tina

Jane, credentialed art therapist, and Tina, her supervisee and art therapy intern, facilitate an open studio weekly in a five-hour window. Located in

DOI: 10.4324/9781003175124-11

an urban medical setting, this studio has a variety of materials available and is open to all inpatients, outpatients, family members, friends, and staff members. A typical studio session is attended by 15 to 20 participants who come and go freely throughout the open studio time frame. Many clients who attend the open studio are receiving comprehensive care from the referring treatment team. Such was the case with Geri who is currently an outpatient client at the hospital.

In Geri's first session, she exhibited an extroverted personality and engaged easily with Jane, Tina, and other studio participants. Her physical appearance was thin, close to emaciation, and her clothing was worn and malodorous. During this, and subsequent sessions, Geri worked closely with Tina. After Geri had been involved in this open studio for several months, she began pushing therapeutic boundaries in a variety of ways. This included arriving shortly before the studio group ended, using/collecting an excessive amount of art supplies, consistently requesting to bring art supplies home with her, not using studio time productively, and impeding on other clients' workspaces. A consistent theme of her work was related to eating, and she frequently discussed difficulties in this area, with Tina and other art therapy clients. For example, she introduced her personal eating preferences to the group and explained that her diet consisted of protein drinks and nutrition bars purchased from the local discount big box store. Tina reported her concerns to Jane, who compiled the information in a report given to the referring treatment team. The treatment team noted the report but no action was taken.

In subsequent open studio sessions, patterns of disordered eating beyond the nutrition bars and protein drinks also emerged. Jane sought consultation with the treatment team regarding concerns with Geri's basic food and shelter needs and discovered that Geri had been neglecting to follow through with treatment team recommendations and referrals. The treatment team informed Jane that Geri had demonstrated a pattern of manipulation. While this information assuaged Jane's concerns, Jane did not share these details with her supervisee Tina.

Geri's eating-related issues continue to worsen to the point where she was admitted to inpatient treatment and given a feeding tube. During Geri's hospitalization, Tina provided in-room art therapy sessions for her. When discharge became imminent, Geri made an attempt to leave with the feeding tube and the police became involved. Unbeknownst to Jane, Tina had provided her personal phone number to Geri, stayed in touch with her, and tried to connect her with social support services. In her efforts, Tina contacted several agencies on Geri's behalf. At the same time, unbeknownst to Tina, the treatment team had made efforts to provide Geri with social support and case management services. Complicating things further, Tina did not inform Jane that she had provided support to Geri outside of the open studio sessions.

11.2 Analysis of the Case

While art therapy supervisors are obligated to provide education and facilitate professional growth, they also play a gatekeeping role and need to ensure client well-being. In this case, Jane has discovered that, due to a breakdown in communication, Tina has unknowingly taken on an inappropriate role in treatment, which has led to Tina potentially practicing outside of her education, training, and competence. This is problematic according to ATCB (2021) code 1.3.3 and American Art Therapy Association (2013) principle 8.3.

11.2.1 D-Dilemma

As Jane considers potential courses of action, two possibilities emerge. Option One is to report the situation to the treatment team, Tina's art therapy training program, and terminate the supervision relationship. Option Two is to connect Tina to the treatment team and allow her to contribute to the team's comprehensive treatment plan. This would provide an opportunity for Tina to learn about working in teams and making appropriate referrals.

To visually process this dilemma, Jane creates a collage depicting two forms of supervision (see Figure 11.1). In the upper right corner, a scene demonstrates the supervisee exploring independently with their back toward the two supervisors who are not focused on the supervisee figure. Angels dance on the opposite side of the upper portion. On the lower side of the collage exists an encapsulated parent and child. This representation reflects a more direct supervision model involving instruction, and teaching techniques. Other elements of the collage include a base representing food and shelter which were the issues the intern was trying to assist with, and a human heart in the center to remind of the human necessity for differing supervision styles.

11.2.1.1 Option One: Codes and Principles Supporting Option One

Option One involves reporting the situation to the treatment team, Tina's art therapy training program, and terminating the supervision relationship due to an inappropriate role that Tina has assumed with Geri. This option is supported by several codes and principles. Code 1.3.3 of the Art Therapy Credentials Board indicates that supervisors need to prevent supervisees from engaging in practices outside of their scope of competence (ATCB, 2021). Likewise, American Art Therapy Association (2013) principle 8.3 specifies that supervisors need to ensure supervisees are not

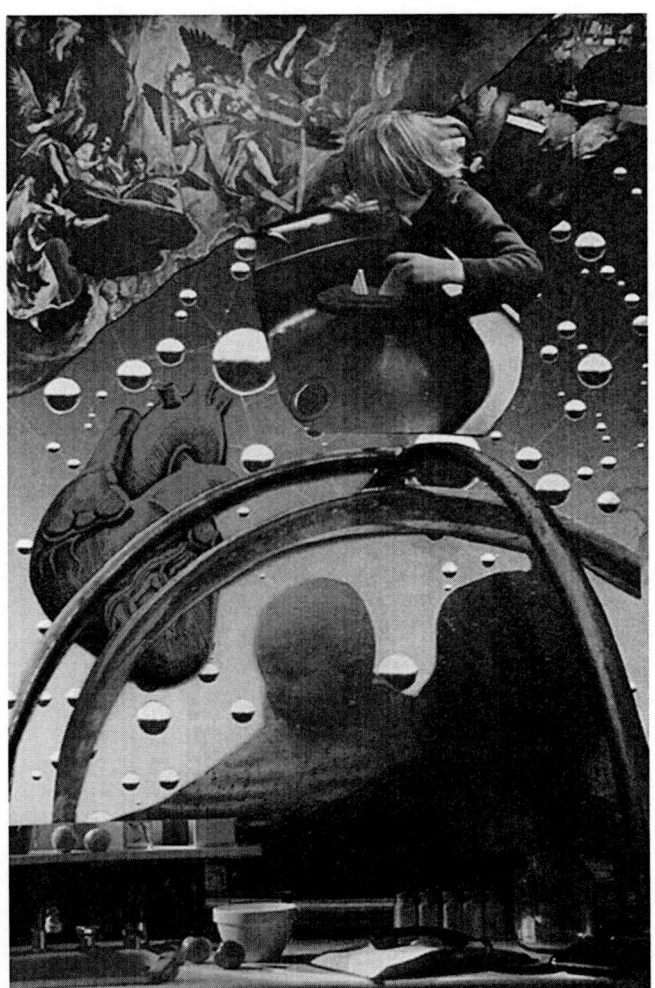

Figure 11.1 Collage revealing supervision styles.

practicing outside their scope of training or expertise. In this situation, Tina is clearly stepping outside of her scope of competence and Jane needs to take steps to remedy this situation immediately. By removing Tina from the situation and the unofficial role of a case manager, Jane is abiding by principle 1.3, which speaks to avoiding ambiguity in roles (American Art Therapy Association, 2013). She is also simultaneously supporting the ideas of beneficence and nonmaleficence because Geri will no longer be receiving inappropriate support from Tina.

11.2.1.2 Option One: Codes and Principles Discouraging Option One

Although there are codes and principles that support removing Tina from the situation, there are also codes and principles that discourage this option. ATCB (2021) code 1.3.1 indicates part of the supervisor's responsibility is fostering the professional growth of the student intern. In this situation, removing Tina would not afford her an opportunity for that growth. In addition, ATCB (2021) code 1.3.7.3 explains the importance of making sure Tina is educated in ethical codes and principles; removing her would preclude her learning from this ethical situation. This option would also deny Tina the opportunity to seek further evaluation and feedback, which is a supervisor responsibility identified in ATCB (2021) code 1.3.7.5.

11.2.1.3 Option Two: Codes and Principles Supporting Option Two

Option Two involves establishing a relationship between Tina and the treatment team (including various case managers). This option would support Tina's desire to stay on track to join the field of art therapy, allow her to clarify roles, and save her potential embarrassment. By including Tina, Jane upholds ATCB (2021) code 1.3.1, which suggests that fostering professional development is among the responsibilities of the supervisor. In addition, Jane has a duty to uphold ATCB (2021) code 1.3.7.3 underscoring art therapists' needs to support the education of ethical standards for supervisees. Allowing Tina to participate in the treatment team's actions going forward would also support her learning the practice and traditions of cooperating fields as expected by ATCB (2021) code 2.3.10.

11.2.1.4 Option Two: Codes and Principles Discouraging Option Two

There are also codes and principles that discourage Tina's participation with the treatment team. ATCB (2021) code 1.3.3 states that "art therapists must not permit students… to perform or represent themselves as competent to perform professional services beyond their education…" (p. 4). Letting Tina work with the treatment team runs the risk of further blurring the roles and responsibilities of art therapists. This would also align with principle 1.3 addressing avoiding ambiguity in roles (American Art Therapy Association, 2013). Finally, American Art Therapy Association (2013) principle 8.3 needs to be considered in this option because the student intern does not have the appropriate experience and education to participate fully in the treatment team.

11.2.2 O-Outcomes

In this case, the relevant parties are Tina, Jane, Geri, and the treatment team (including the case managers). In both options, there are impacts to each of these parties.

11.2.2.1 Option One

A breach in the scope of practice has occurred and the treatment team will need to work towards a solution. If Jane were to remove Tina from the situation, Tina would be excluded from playing a role in remedying the situation and would miss out on valuable learning opportunities regarding treatment team cooperation. Jane would address the situation with the treatment team in order to engage in problem-solving around the needs of the client. The relationship between Jane, Tina, and her training program could be strained and limit opportunities for future art therapy interns from that program. Undesirably, Jane would be placed in a situation where she would be remedying a situation that Tina contributed to, without Tina.

Geri will also be impacted through the dissolution of the therapy relationship with Tina. Regardless of whether Geri experienced Tina as an art therapy resource, a consoling friend, or a means to an end, the relationship would be dismantled. This option would also not further Tina's education in rapport building, desirable relational dynamics, or attempts at appropriate mutual termination.

11.2.2.2 Option Two

If Option Two is selected, Tina begins building a relationship with the treatment team, and works with the case manager to establish appropriate referrals for the client. Tina would be directed to communicate the events and her unintentional misstep directly to the case manager and treatment team. Ideally, Geri's case will be reviewed, and Tina will be able to understand how different practitioners contribute to client care. Tina benefits from this option through experiential learning across a professional spectrum. This option may cause distress for Tina in anticipation of disclosing the situation to the treatment team. Jane would have to support and supervise Tina throughout the process of implementing Option Two. At the same time, Jane would need to relinquish some control over Tina's training process since the treatment team would now be playing a more active role in supervision. There is also the potential for additional work as Jane may need to re-negotiate art therapy internship agreements with the training program. Geri may benefit from the continued relationship with Tina in that it would model healthy relationship-building and interdisciplinary treatment approaches. Working with Geri could also become a learning opportunity for Tina, and this may deepen Tina's understanding and self-awareness with regard to manipulation and effective boundaries in relationships.

The case manager and treatment team are also impacted by incorporating Tina into their workload. The case manager will need to take time to bring Tina up to date with client treatment schedules and the treatments and services that have been incorporated into Geri's care. While the workload for the case manager may increase, this would allow the case manager and treatment team to explore this case from the perspective of a student intern.

11.2.3 A-Assistance

11.2.3.1 Assistance from Consultants: Legal

Three resources have been identified as valuable consultants for legal questions in this case. The medical director of the clinic where the art therapists are employed, the system legal department, and the school's clinical coordinator. The questions for the medical director might be, are there system policies and/or procedures regarding referrals? And are there reporting standards that this would fall under and need reporting? The medical director is likely to say there are system policies in place and these documented procedures lend support towards Option Two. Jane would be able to show and engage the student intern in the procedure rather than explaining from a passive perspective. Jane may also ask: does the contract between the school and the site allow the student to join non-art therapy-based treatment professionals in practice? This answer could vary between schools and highlights the attention that must be paid regarding art therapy practice and client contact limitations.

11.2.3.2 Assistance from Consultants: Ethical

The treatment team is another valuable consultant in this case. Three questions the art therapists may have for them are: what is the impact on the role of the case manager? Are there other practices and standards that need to be considered? What is the scope of practice of an art therapist in regard to referrals based upon a membership on this treatment team? It is likely that the student's interference undermined the established relationship between the client and the treatment team. Indeed, the art therapists should have referred the client to the case manager for basic human needs. These answers both support Option Two and suggest the importance of remedial supervision for the student intern by the art therapist.

11.2.3.3 Assistance from Consultants: Clinical

One question an art therapist may have regarding the clinical implications of the situation is: could there be ramifications for the client beyond our current understanding of the situation? For instance, could there be a hidden agenda behind the manipulative nature of the client? This question would be most appropriate for a clinician who specializes in cancer care. The clinician is likely to say the client's behavior may be indicative of a mental health challenge involving hoarding and emotional manipulation of others and this lends support towards Option Two. Relevant factors in implementing Option Two and preventing future issues include informing students to not share personal contact information with clients, teaching them how to maintain time structures and boundaries, and keeping interns informed of why boundaries were instituted with their clients.

11.2.3.4 Assistance from Consultants: Risk Management

With regard to risk management, a question for the medical director is, are there ramifications for this department or for the larger system? To minimize risks, this situation needs to be addressed and caution needs to be taken to avoid similar incidents from occurring. A question for an expert clinician is, are there dangers for the client if the out-of-scope referrals are followed up with? If the client uses unofficial referrals, the treatment team would not be able to coordinate care. The answers to these questions support Option One which removes the student intern from the situation.

11.2.3.5 Assistance from the Literature

The literature relevant to this situation identifies three areas of concern that need to be considered: scope of practice, supervision for remediation, and adequacy of supervision. With regard to the scope of practice, Beyene et al. (2019) defined professional boundaries in light of dignified mental health care. Berggren and Severinsson (2006) explored a similar framework around supervision in recognizing the integration of team cooperation, patient relations, and feelings toward patients. Student interns in various professions need to first ensure safety, empower, and build integrity. This happens through the integration of theoretical knowledge and finding substance in their chosen profession. In parallel fashion, Beyene et al. (2019) found three themes present in maintaining client autonomy in shared decision making: recognition of value and expressed knowledge of the case, approaching with awareness of comprehension of circumstances, and responding from a place grounded in acknowledgment. These themes also reflect the approaches of supervisors to supervisees in developing competence (Berggren & Severinsson, 2006). Taken together, these sources provide support for Option Two because engagement with the treatment team would provide teaching opportunities and allow the intern further professional development.

With regard to supervision for remediation, Thomas (2014) explains the causes and types of ethical violations where supervision may be a remedy. Specifically, potential causes for transgressions include ignorance or lack of knowledge, countertransference, and the assumption that exceptions would exist for a given client. Thomas (2014) suggests supervisors recognize and discuss four areas with their supervisees: (1) a realistic conceptualization of the situation, (2) an examination of both actual and potential impacts, (3) a generalized understanding comparing the case to a compliant case, and (4) identify warning signs that may have indicated the transgression of boundaries. If defensiveness prevents remediation through supervision, the gatekeeping role of the supervisor may become prioritized. Throughout the progress of remedial supervision, it is important for the supervisor to remember "no one is invulnerable to making mistakes" (Thomas, 2014, p. 1112). This resource supports Option Two if Tina is open to remediation but supports Option One if she is not.

Finally, in the area of adequate supervision, Ellis et al. (2014) defined harmful supervision versus inadequate supervision by establishing a list of minimum standards for adequate supervision. Interestingly, this study found that inadequate supervision is more common than harmful supervision and it is important to be able to distinguish between the two. By providing Jane with an opportunity to remedy the supervision oversight, she models how to recognize and address inadequate supervision. This supports Tina's professional development and teaches her effective and appropriate strategies for working as a member of a treatment team.

To integrate the assistance received from literature and consultants, Jane created a pen and ink sketch that depicted three levels (see Figure 11.2). The top-level was a medical system, the middle level was a treatment team working around a table, and the bottom level was a student art therapy intern working with a patient in a hospital room. The sketch helped bring awareness to the layers of impact this scope of practice breach could bring to the larger system.

11.2.4 R-Responsibility/Risk

Jane faces potential risks from the client, the art therapy intern, the treatment team, the case manager, and the intern's academic institution. Each option creates exposure to risk and opportunities to fulfill responsibilities with each of the parties.

11.2.4.1 Option One

If Jane removes Tina from the situation, Tina may file a complaint against Jane for inadequate supervision. Tina could interpret the removal as punishment for Jane's mistakes, and may believe her supervisor is not

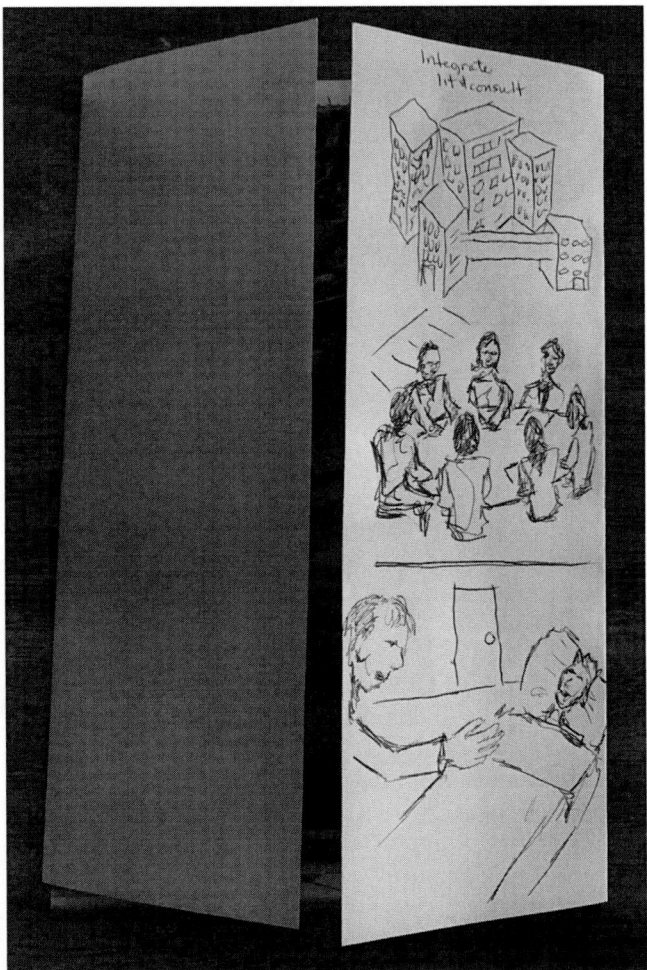

Figure 11.2 Sketch of various levels of treatment.

taking Geri's best interests into consideration. The academic institution may question the appropriateness of removing Tina, and argue that Jane has not fulfilled her responsibility to the academic institution as a site supervisor. However, Geri, the case manager, and the treatment team are less likely to file ethics complaints. With the interdisciplinary nature of the treatment, Geri may not be aware of the situation and assume Tina's removal is part of her training schedule. By following the proper procedures, the art therapist would be fulfilling the responsibility to the treatment team and the case manager, who would likely appreciate the proper procedure being followed to give referrals.

11.2.4.2 Option Two

In Option Two, Jane may have some risk with the treatment team, specifically the case manager. While Jane would be providing an educational opportunity and help Tina network with the team, integrating a new provider would create more work for the team and case manager. Geri would be unaffected because her treatment would continue. Tina would be given an opportunity to grow as a professional, learn about working within a treatment team, and how to properly follow the referral procedure process. Jane would be treating Tina as a professional colleague who is capable of working with others to remedy her mistakes. Presuming the supervision agreement allows, the academic institution would likely approve of the educational opportunity afforded to the student intern.

11.2.5 T-Take Action

After analyzing the case of Geri and Tina, Option Two seems like the most ethical option. Option Two is supported by ATCB (2021) code 1.3.1, 1.3.7.3, and 2.3.10. In addition, Option Two has positive impacts on the growth of the student intern, because they are able to learn experientially about the treatment team and how professionals can intersect in a respectful and professional manner. Option Two is also supported by recent literature which provides a venue for remediation (e.g., Thomas, 2014), and supervisor development (e.g., Ellis et al., 2014). In taking Option Two, the art therapist minimizes risk from the student intern who will be offered the opportunity to explore and re-address boundary transgressions both with clients and other professions.

Jane revisits her original collage and finds that Option Two is represented closer to the exploratory end of the supervision spectrum (see Figure 11.1). While this option requires the student to work collaboratively with other members of the treatment team, it also allows an expansion of the intern's education beyond the scope of art therapy and supports learning about related professions.

11.3 Summary of the Main Concerns

The main concerns in ensuring adequate supervision include: (1) communication between the supervisor and supervisee, (2) issues regarding the scope of practice, and (3) the importance of the supervisory relationship along with supervisory style. Clear communication between supervisors and supervisees minimizes the risk. Scope of practice violation is another primary concern, relevant to all supervisors. Supervisors are tasked with monitoring and ensuring supervisees do not practice outside their scope of competence. The alignment of supervision styles is also important for ensuring a successful supervision experience. People learn in diverse ways: some require visual information, some learn best from reading, while others respond better from being told information. A mismatch in supervision and learning styles can result in consequences ranging from ineffective communication to ethical violations.

11.4 Tips for Avoiding Pitfalls

To prevent ethical missteps in supervision, art therapy supervisors should enhance their own education regarding supervision. Further, adapting the supervision style being used to the needs of the supervisee may be beneficial. Moreover, supervisors should remember to keep supervisees informed when following through with concerns about clients.

Creating an onboarding process that teaches supervisees about the referral process, the work of the entire treatment team, and the art therapist's role among that team can be beneficial. Indeed, supervisees should be aware of the collaborative nature of treatment and being familiar with the members of a treatment team before working with clients would be advantageous. With an understanding of who makes up the treatment team and their roles, supervisees may be more adept at working within their own scope of practice and following proper protocol for referring to other professionals.

11.5 Suggested Further Readings

Abrams, R. & Nolan, E. (2016). Developing a master's student's research and practitioner skills through collaboration with a doctoral researcher. *Art Therapy: Journal of the American Art Therapy Association, 33*(1), 46–50. https://doi.org/10.1080/07421656.2016.1127615

This article articulates the importance of the development of a supervisory relationship that includes awareness of the student's readiness. Establishing the supervisory relationship paralleled the building of relationships with clients including understanding and practice within an evidence base. Grasping the scope and readiness of a master's student's understanding and engagement in research and practice supports the supervisor's role in mentorship. The attuned supervisory relationship increased the master's student's efficacy in professional art therapy relationships.

Deaver, S. P., & Shiflett, C. (2011). Art-based supervision techniques. *Art Therapy: Journal of the American Art Therapy Association, 30*(2), 257–276. https://doi.org/10.1080/07325223.2011.619456

This article highlights the importance of clinical supervision in the development of an art therapy master's student. It encourages reflective practice regarding client relationships along with art-based measures to highlight and mirror creative processes. The focus on learning through clinical art therapy supervision is seen as strengthened by student engagement as opposed to following directive lesson plans. The article emphasizes the strength of artmaking in client conceptualization in art therapy.

Fish, B. (2016). *Art-based Supervision: Cultivating insight through imagery.* Routledge. https://doi.org/10.4324/9781315747538

Response art, created by a clinician and/or student clinician, allows an in-depth review of client circumstances through the lens of the therapeutic relationship. Response art reveals layers of understanding regarding clients and in turn, understanding between supervisor and supervisee in art-based supervision. Fish introduces a phenomenon she calls Harm's Touch focused on the impact of trauma within the clinical and supervisory relationships. This book also addresses hierarchical power differentials that exist within the supervisory relationship.

Goodyear, R., Lichtenberg, J. W., Bang, K., & Gragg, J. B. (2014). Ten changes psychotherapists typically make as they mature into the role of supervisor. *Journal of Clinical Psychology: In Session, 70*(11), 1042–1050. https://doi.org/10.1002/jclp.22125

Goodyear et al. (2014) explored the development of mental health supervisors based upon Heid's 10 projected dimensions. The dimensions were scaled and edited by seven expert supervisors and explained as developmental events. These events included the ability to perceive and act on complex situations, a growing identity as a supervisor, the ability to be one's self in practice, seeing one's self as a supervisor, being able to use reflection as a tool to manage bias and projections, confidence in judgment, confidence in competence, finding patience with supervisee's level of development, courage in the gatekeeping role, and the ability to conceptualize and incorporate power.

Miller, A. (2012). Inspired by El Duende: One-canvas process painting in art therapy supervision. *Art Therapy: Journal of the American Art Therapy Association, 29*(4), 166–173. http://doi.org/10.1080/07421656.2013.730024

Miller describes a balance between excess and dearth of didactic instruction. Her experience defines an ongoing painting process done in the style of *El Duende,* this process is seen as incorporating layers of power in reflection that can attune archetypal, clinical, and personal experiences. The layered painting is seen as the student's voice and becomes central to the supervisory relationship. Examples provided demonstrate symbolic dialog and tensions inherent within the painting process. Through the *El Duende* process, students developed awareness in conceptualization, and therapeutic presence.

Tangen, J. L. (2018). Learning styles and supervision: A clinical review. *The Clinical Review: In Session, 70*(11), 241–256. https://doi.org/10.1080/07325223.2017.1388897

Tangen (2018) evaluated learning styles in relation to supervision. Tangen noted that supervisees learning styles often change through the trajectory of learning where supervision styles are often constant per supervisor. It was noted that best practices in supervision include consideration and implementation of learning styles although there is very little established evidence of its effectiveness. Tangen recommends situational awareness of limitations, consideration of intentions of both supervisor and supervisees styles, and awareness of any psychometrics and evidence of any models being used.

References

American Art Therapy Association. (2013). *Ethical principles for art therapists.* http://www.arttherapy.org/upload/ethicalprinciples.pdf

Art Therapy Credentials Board. (2021). *Code of professional practice.* https://www. atcb.org/resource/pdf/ATCB-Code-of-Ethics-Conduct-DisciplinaryProcedures.pdf

Barnett, J. E., & Molzon, C. H. (2014). Clinical supervision of psychotherapy: Essential ethics issues for supervisors and supervisees. *Journal of Clinical Psychology, 70*(11), 1051–1061. 10.1002/jclp.22126

Berggren, I., & Severinsson, E. (2006). The significance of nurse supervisors' different ethical decision-making styles. *Journal of Nurse Management, 14*(8), 637–643. 10.1111/j.1365-2934.2006.00710.x

Beyene, L. S., Severinsson, E., Hansen, B. S., & Rortveit, K. (2019). Being in a space of shared decision-making for dignified mental care. *Journal of Psychiatric and Mental Health Nursing, 26*(9/10), 368–376. 10.1111/jpm.12548

Carrigan, J. (1993). Ethical considerations in a supervisory relationship: A synthesis. *Art Therapy: Journal of the American Art Therapy Association, 10*(3), 130–135. 10.1080/07421656.1993.10758997

Ellis, M. V., Berger, L., Hanus, A. E., Ayala, E. E., Swords, B. A., & Siembor, M. (2014). Inadequate and harmful clinical supervision: Testing a revised framework and assessing occurrence. *The Counseling Psychologist, 42*(4), 434–472. 10.1177/0011000013508656

Goodyear, R., Lichtenberg, J. W., Bang, K., & Gragg, J. B. (2014). Ten changes psychotherapists typically make as they mature into the role of supervisor. *Journal of Clinical Psychology, 70*(11), 1042–1050. 10.1002/jclp.22125

Kurpius, D., & Gibson, G. (1991). Ethical issues in supervising counseling practitioners. *Counseling Education & Supervision, 31*(1), 48–55. 10.1002/j.1556-6978.1991.tb00370.x

Tangen, J. L. (2018). Learning styles and supervision: A clinical review. *The Clinical Supervisor, 37*(2), 241–256. 10.1080/07325223.2017.1388897

Thomas, J. T. (2014). Disciplinary supervision following ethics complaint: Goals, tasks, and ethical dimensions. *Journal of Clinical Psychology, 70*(11), 1104–1114. 10.1002/jclp.22131

12 Ethics in Research: A Case of Misunderstanding, Fabrication, & Plagiarism

Patricia A. St John Tager

Research ethics is directly addressed by many professional fields. In art therapy, five ethical values are identified: Autonomy, Beneficence, Nonmaleficence, Justice, Fidelity, and Veracity (Farrant et al., 2014, p. 13). Similarly, the National Institutes of Health (2021) Clinical Center lists the following ethical guidelines: social and clinical value, scientific validity, fair subject selection, favorable risk-benefit ratio, independent review, informed consent, and respect for potential and enrolled subjects. Relevant discussions of research ethics within the broad field of mental health are found in numerous publications. For example, Corts and Tatum (2019) observe that ethics should be examined from the perspective of the researcher's values, but that all ethical behaviors in research are based on honesty, accuracy, efficiency, and objectivity.

In art therapy, research ethics are identified in ethical codes by the two major art therapy associations: the American Art Therapy Association (AATA) Ethical Principles for Art Therapists (2013) and the Art Therapy Credentials Board (ATCB) Code of Ethics, Conduct, and Disciplinary Procedures (2021). Several codes and principles are relevant to the ethical practice of research with human participants. These include confidentiality, professional competence and integrity, and responsibility to the profession. Research ethics is also addressed in various art therapy publications. For example, Betts and Deaver (2019) discuss research with vulnerable populations, using artwork in research, and the importance of Institutional Review Boards (IRB). Likewise, Kapitan (2018) discusses multiple roles, confidentiality and anonymity, informed consent, deception, and disclosure in research.

When translated to practice, these guidelines result in specific practices that are considered violations of research ethics. For example, the federal Office of Science and Technology identifies fabrication, falsification, and plagiarism under the definition of research misconduct and explains that such misconduct may undermine public trust in research findings and their application (Columbia University, n.d.). Indeed, Daniel-McKeigue (2007) argues that maintaining high values is the driving force behind ethical research behaviors. Consequently, it is important to consider that

DOI: 10.4324/9781003175124-12

while research may be conducted in an academic setting, its findings and application transcend the traditional academic boundaries. In summary, research ethics have far-reaching implications.

12.1 The Case of Sophia and Kayla

Sophia (a pseudonym) has been a full-time assistant professor and program director at a small, private liberal arts college, administrating and teaching in the master's degree program in art therapy. She is well-liked and respected by colleagues, staff, and administrators. Among the many courses, she teaches are those in research methodology and thesis which are taken in sequence by students during their final semesters. She has taught these two courses for 10 years and mentored many thesis studies.

Her graduate student, Kayla, attends full-time and is near graduation. While research was a new area for Kayla and she struggled to fully understand some assignments, she passed the research methodology course but barely earned a grade of "B." During the course, Kayla identified a thesis project, wrote a review of related literature, and planned her thesis research study to be conducted in the next semester.

Sophia's fall semester research class requires students to propose, conduct, and write up a study suitable for the Institutional Review Board's (IRB) assessment and approval. Students are aware of the time constraints and as such plan projects that fit into a 15-week semester. Since proposals often require revision, student researchers are asked to factor in this possibility. During the first two weeks of the semester the IRB reviews and approves or disapproves every research study in time to allow students to conduct their studies during the next 10 to 11 weeks. In the final weeks of the course, students finish writing their theses and present them publicly. This course is one of the last steps students take prior to graduation.

Research is a new area for Kayla, as it is for many students whose undergraduate major did not require empirical research. She enrolled in the thesis course ready to submit her proposal to the IRB. She planned to conduct a single-subject study using an A-B-A format. Her hypothesis is that participants will spend more time-on-task during sensory-based art therapy sessions than during art-therapy-as-usual, which consists of directives and highly structured treatment sessions. Kayla's proposal indicates she will conduct the study at her internship site, a pre-school where she has a good working relationship with the children and her supervisor, Gabrielle.

The thesis course is configured to provide ongoing back-and-forth feedback between the instructor and students. Students are invited to share problems that inevitably arise and problem-solve solutions with classmates and the instructor. A few weeks into the course, Sophia notices that Kayla's contributions are very brief and have little detail. While Kayla seems enthusiastic about the treatment sessions and says the children are enjoying them, she does not talk about typical obstacles and challenges that often occur when conducting a research study with children, such as having difficulty obtaining parental consent. As the semester progresses, Sophia reminds the class of the importance of attention to these details and the time frame for completing their studies.

A unique aspect of the course is that students are allowed to review past, completed theses as examples of content and formatting. Kayla selects a thesis study based on a single-subject methodology on a topic very similar to hers. As the semester nears the end, Sophia continues to be concerned that Kayla's contributions lack detail and specificity. Surprisingly, in the final class presentation, Kayla provides detailed data and a thorough final paper, which includes a specific and insightful discussion. All of this is a marked improvement from her earlier submissions.

Sophia finds this concerning and asks Kayla to meet with her during office hours. She also emails Gabrielle and is surprised to learn that Gabrielle is unaware that Kayla planned to conduct a study at the site. Sophia compares Kayla's submitted results and discussion chapters to the single-subject example thesis available to the class. She discovers that Kayla appears to have plagiarized significant portions of the example thesis, including text and tables, while only changing the data slightly.

At their meeting, Sophia confronts Kayla about her observations and concerns regarding plagiarism and fabrication. Kayla responds by saying:

> I gave the children six sensory-based lessons, the lessons in my presentation and written thesis. I didn't know I was supposed to carry out the study. I thought it was just an exercise, a practice or pretend study, like we did in class last semester.

Kayla explains she did not mean to break rules and just wanted the assignment to be done so she could graduate next month. Sophia explains to Kayla that she misunderstood the assignment and that she not only had to work with the children but also conduct the study. She was required to obtain parental consent, train an observer to gather data, and analyze the data. Sophia goes on to explain that this constitutes fabrication because the proposed study did not occur. Sophia also brings up the problem of plagiarism and shows Kayla the chapters, side-by-side. Sophia points out the similarities and, in many places, exactly the same wording, tables, and slightly altered data.

In alignment with professional organizations, the College's Academic Integrity statement identifies fabricating and plagiarism as violations that carry penalties. However, Sophia is troubled because on one hand she understands what happened and feels the need to rescue Kayla from this appalling situation; on the other hand, she wonders whether she might have contributed to Kayla's misunderstanding by not catching the problem earlier in the semester.

Sophia recalls that Kayla never previously fabricated or plagiarized, and maintained a GPA of 3.0. However, Sophia is very concerned about Kayla's misunderstanding of the assignment and how she handled it. Given the circumstances, that Kayla was at the end of the program, Sophia initially considers just disregarding the situation, as some professors do when they have little to no evidence of ethical misconduct (Hard et al., 2006; Keith-Spiegel et al., 2010). However, because Kayla has admitted to research misconduct, Sophia must determine whether Kayla should be given a chance to rectify her infraction. One option would be to grant Kayla an extension to conduct the study, which would delay her graduation to August instead of May, but still allow her to participate in the May commencement exercises. Another option would be for Sophia to respond to the seriousness of the infraction, provide a grade of "F" for the course, and enforce the college's requirement to retake the course.

12.2 Analysis of the Case

Sophia has two options. She could opt for containment of the infractions by entering a grade of "Incomplete" rather than a grade of "F", extend the time for Kayla to actually carry out the study, and rewrite the remaining chapters. This route requires Kayla to return to the site, pending Gabrielle's consent, and conduct the study. In Option Two, strictly following the college's academic integrity requirements, a grade of "F" is entered. Kayla re-takes the course when it is subsequently offered. For both options, a report of the violations would be submitted to the associate dean and become part of Kayla's permanent record.

12.2.1 D-Dilemma

In addition to the college's policies and procedures and to help her with her deliberations, Sophia checks the American Art Therapy Association's Ethical Principles for Art Therapists (2013) and the Art Therapy Credentials Board's (2021) *Code of Ethics, Conduct, and Disciplinary Procedures* to determine which policies are applicable. To help her process the options, Sophia creates an abstract image representing the dilemma (Figure 12.1). It captures her confusion, agitated mood, the sensation of coming unraveled, and emptiness at her core depicting her feelings of aloneness.

12.2.1.1 Option One: Codes Principles Supporting Option One

In Option One, Sophia would enter a grade of "Incomplete", allow Kayla to conduct the study during the summer, and upon submission of the thesis and presentation enter a letter grade. The college's academic

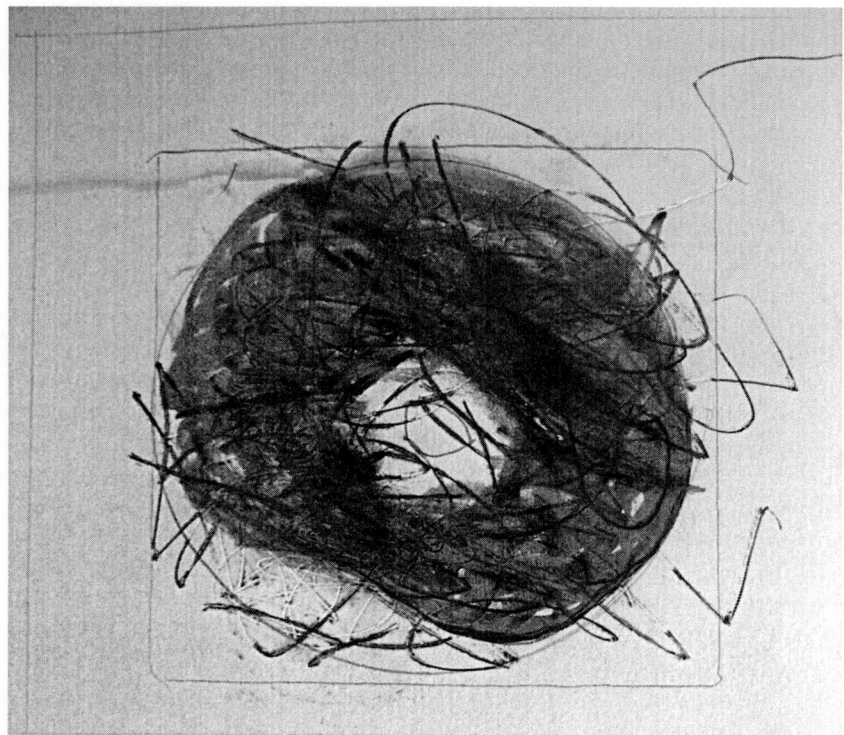

Figure 12.1 Dilemma – Confusion, trying to hold together, but "at loose ends."

integrity policy and procedures list penalties for academic dishonesty, including fabrication and plagiarism but also allows a faculty member to provide a reasonable opportunity for a student to resubmit an assignment after admitting to an alleged infraction.

Option One is supported by Art Therapy Credentials Board (2021) 1.3.7.5, under Responsibility to Students and Supervisees, regarding providing adequate responses to students' weekly posts and in-class reports. Sophia kept written records of Kayla's progress and supported her throughout the semester. She gave regular feedback to Kayla in class and on thesis sections submitted by Kayla. Allowing for Kayla to resubmit her work would continue this feedback and evaluation process.

Option One is also supported by ATCB 1.3.7.3, which states that art therapists and, in this case, art therapy educators, make students aware of current ethical standards. By confronting Kayla and offering an incomplete for the class, Sophia can use this situation as an educational experience.

12.2.1.2 Option One: Codes and Principles Discouraging Option One

The American Art Therapy Association's (AATA, 2013) principle 8.1 specifies that research and results need to be accurate and of high quality. By downplaying the plagiarism and fabrication and allowing Kayla to complete her study, Sophia does not uphold the high caliber of research expected in art therapy. Further, AATA principle 9.1 emphasizes the necessity of following research protocols and these protocols do not include fabricating results and then re-conducting a study. Further, American Art Therapy Association (2013) principle 8.3 and ATCB (2021) code 1.3.3 indicate that art therapists do not let students present themselves as competent when they are not. By minimizing the research ethics infraction, Sophia may be furthering Kayla's misrepresentation of her competence level.

12.2.1.3 Option Two: Codes and Principles Supporting Option Two

Option Two, assign a failing grade, is supported by the college's academic integrity policies and procedures. The implications of this are that Kayla would be required to retake the course in the next academic year and delay her degree conferral.

Option Two is also supported by ATCB (2021) code 2.7, regarding documenting information required by the institution. By assigning a failing grade, Sophia would memorialize the research ethics infraction. ATCB code 1.4, regarding research participants, institutional review board approvals, and other requirements when conducting research also support Option Two. Left unaddressed, this research ethics infraction would not fulfill obligations to research participants. American Art Therapy Association (2013) principle 8.1, and ATCB (2021) code 1.3.2 further support Option Two by specifying that art therapy educators ensure and uphold high standards with students and supervisees. Sophia failing Kayla ensures that these professional standards are met. Likewise, it is supported by American Art Therapy Association (2013) principle 10.8 because the failing grade prevents these fabricated results from being released widely.

12.2.1.4 Option Two: Codes and Principles Discouraging Option Two

ATCB (2021) code 1.3.7.5 specifies that art therapist supervisors give students adequate feedback. Failing Kayla does not allow Sophia to provide feedback in a way that promotes growth. Likewise, ATCB code 1.3.1 states that art therapists foster the growth of students and advisees; but, by failing Kayla, Sophia eliminates this opportunity. Finally, the

American Art Therapy Association (2013) aspirational ethical principle of autonomy discourages failing Kayla as it does not allow her the opportunity to rectify her research ethics error and, instead, makes the decision on how to solve the misstep for her.

12.2.2 O-Outcomes

The relevant parties in this dilemma are Sophia, Kayla, her classmates, Gabrielle, the potential research participants, and the college. She again turns to art making to assist in identifying her options and their subsequent outcomes. The image she creates has a movable paper divider which she uses to weigh the options (see Figure 12.2). The left Option is open to suggestions, receiving outside sources' recommendations, and taking in information. It perfectly balances the right side Option which is similar to the "Dilemma" drawing, except that the unraveling lines are now tightly bound in the middle. Unlike Figure 12.1 – Dilemma where the center is empty; the right side of Figure 12.2 – Options is dark, closed, and impenetrable.

12.2.2.1 Option One

If Option One is taken, Kayla has the opportunity to conduct the study honestly and in compliance with the College's policies and those of the AATA and ATCB. However, this does obligate Gabrielle and the potential study participants to work with Kayla beyond the originally agreed-upon timeframe. While Kayla's infractions will be on the record, the consequences are less impactful on Kayla's progression toward becoming a credentialed art therapist. Further, Sophia and the college adhere to the flexibility in the Academic Integrity policy.

However, providing Kayla with an incomplete for the course creates a precedent for future offenses that might conflict with the College's Statement of Academic Integrity. This might result in future students engaging in research ethics violations. Moreover, Sophia could be held responsible by the College for not upholding professional responsibilities and inappropriately allowing Kayla to have a chance to rectify the situation and graduate.

12.2.2.2 Option Two

By entering a grade of "F" for the thesis, Sophia is in compliance with the college's academic integrity statement regarding grading assignments that are in violation to receive a failing grade. However, Kayla's degree conferral would be delayed until such time that she could retake and pass the course.

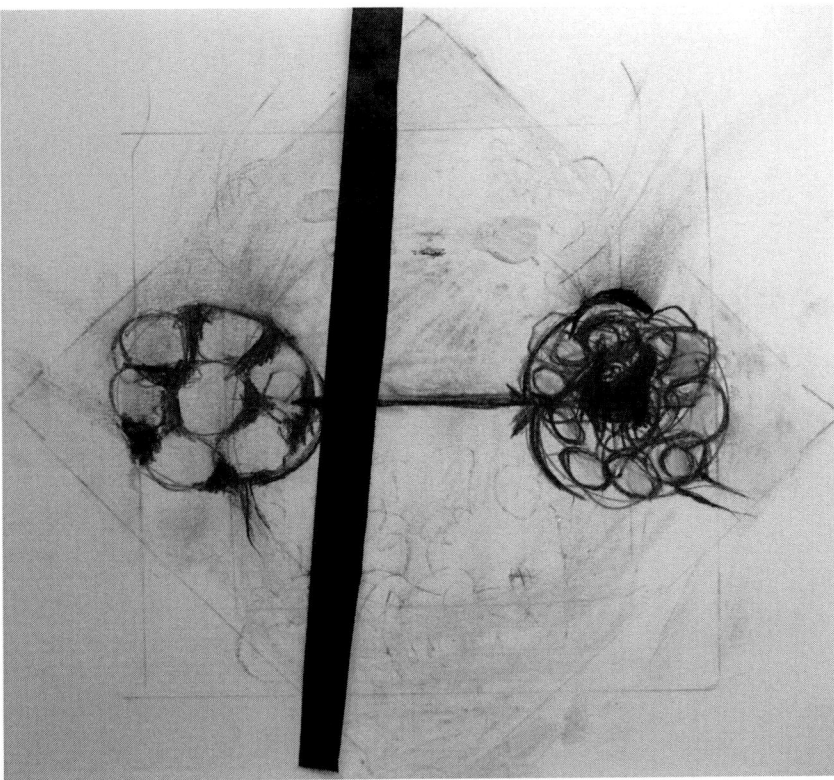

Figure 12.2 Outcomes – Two balls pull at each other. A pendulum vacillates between them.

Further, Gabrielle and the potential study participants would not be pressured to continue involvement with Kayla beyond the agreed-upon timeframe. Likewise, the college would not be placed in a situation where it had to make the determination of whether applying flexibility in the academic integrity statement was appropriate. Finally, other students in the program would not feel that undue special treatment had occurred with Kayla and that all students were held to the same professional standards and expectations.

12.2.3 A-Assistance

To further analyze the situation, Kayla consults with colleagues about their experience with fabrication and plagiarism, and she searches the literature for similar dilemmas. This is consistent with American Art Therapy Association (2013) principle 1.7 which specifies reaching out for

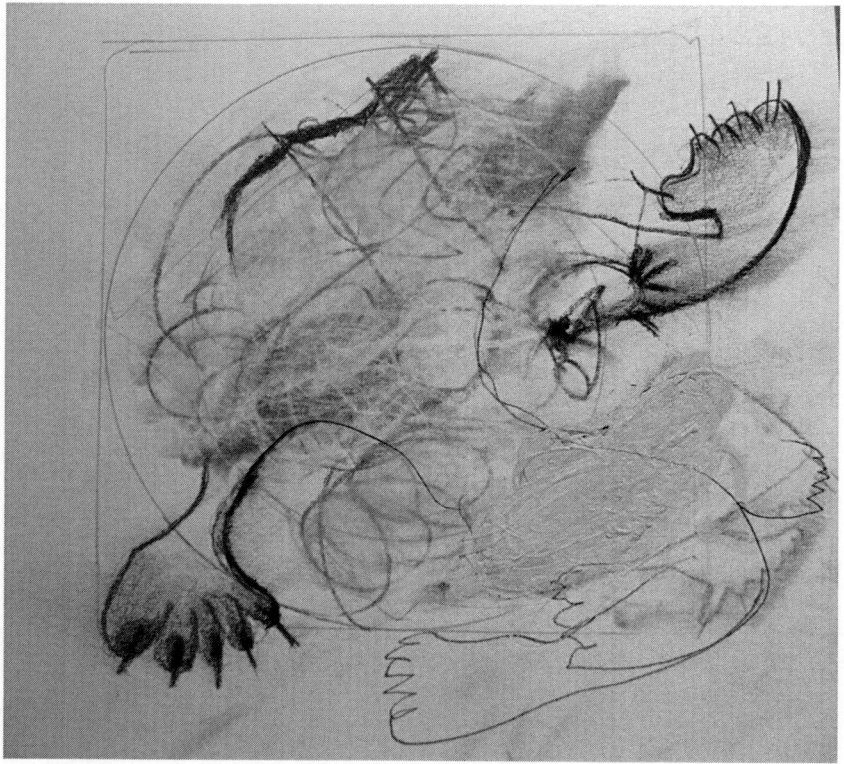

Figure 12.3 Assistance – Hands reach out in search of help.

assistance when challenging situations arise. Sophia's "Assistance" drawing (Figure 12.3) depicts a vague, formless middle and two arms reaching out on the left and right sides, in similar positions to the balls depicted in Figure 12.2 – Options. However, there is more movement in this drawing than is seen in drawings completed during previous steps. Even as the arms reach out, they seem to be paddling in a counter-clockwise direction, suggesting turning back in time and reconsidering.

12.2.3.1 Assistance from Consultants

Sophia enlists several consultants to help her sort out the best option. The first consultant is a trusted colleague who has administered a graduate art therapy program for over 30 years and has experience with cases of fabrication and plagiarism. Sophia asks whether she might be culpable for Kayla's violation of ethical behavior and is told that she would be required to uphold high standards and expect students to abide by the ethical standards of the college, AATA, and ATCB. Consequently, Sophia has a responsibility to identify and censor irresponsible actions, misuse of documents, and reports of false data and results from research studies. Her colleague also explains that Sophia is responsible to ensure course requirements are known to students and students' progress provided. This information would seem to suggest that Sophia should assign a failing grade for Kayla because it would allow her to follow-through on adhering to her various responsibilities.

Sophia also consults with a colleague who teaches ethics and serves on the college's Academic Grievance Committee. Sophia asks historically what has been the outcome when, at the end of their program, a student plagiarizes and fabricates in a required course. Sophia's colleague informs her that there have been a few incidents of this, but when this occurred in a required course, the student re-took the course. This information further supports assigning Kayla a failing grade.

12.2.3.2 Assistance from the Literature

Sophia turns to professional journals where she finds articles on ethical behavior in academic settings. In the first article, Meng et al. (2014) review the literature on reasons and intentions for academic dishonesty using the Theory of Planned Behavior (TPB). This theory posits that academic dishonesty is planned and conscious. It is based on the student's attitude towards academic dishonesty, what the person considers to be the norm for academic dishonesty, and what the person perceives is expected behavior. Expected behaviors are termed "subjective." These three factors are interactive, each one depending on the others to determine whether an act of academic dishonesty will occur.

Related to this theory is an article by Jordan (2010), who conducted a study comparing cheaters with non-cheaters. Information was gathered from each group about what they knew was the college's policy and procedures on cheating, what the participants thought was normative behavior, their own core beliefs, and their level of mastery over the material. Results indicated that cheaters did not cheat in all courses and when they did, it was typically associated with a low level of mastery over the material. Further, there were differences between cheaters and non-cheaters on their perception of normative behavior, understanding of the college's academic honesty policies, and their own core values and beliefs about cheating.

Stearns (2010) found that the relationship between the student and professor affected academic honesty. Specifically, when a professor's behavior was negatively perceived, students were more likely to violate the college's academic honesty policies. In an earlier study, LaBeff et al. (1990) found that 54% of students admitted cheating at least once and justified their behavior as specific to the situation. Finally, Lau and Haug (2011) found that professors' attitudes towards cheating were predictive of cheating, but that students expected faculty members to teach them about what constituted ethical academic behavior and what was unethical.

Hard et al. (2006) found that faculty have an important role in supporting ethical behavior and discouraging violations of academic integrity. Specifically, professors can deter academic dishonesty by consistently confronting students who violate academic integrity policies. Finally, Keith-Spiegel et al. (2010), conducted a study to understand why professors often ignore student academic integrity violations. Professors indicated that lack of evidence, a lack of courage, and avoidance of stress were reasons for not confronting an academically dishonest student. In addition, professors admitted to assuming that students who cheated would be caught at some point or fail a course.

With this information in mind, Sophia feels less alone in her doubts and conflicted emotions. Evidence gleaned from these studies lends support for Option Two. Specifically, that research misconduct is conscious, takes place within the context of the institution's culture, and may be considered "normative" behavior. Within academia, the relationship between students and professors has a bearing on students' decisions to engage in misconduct. Although Keith-Spiegel et al. (2010) note that professors avoid confronting students, it is evident that this evasion is not condoned.

12.2.4 R-Responsibility/Risk

Responsibility/Risk, the next step in the DO ART process, includes potential risks facing Sophia from Kayla, Gabrielle, the potential participants, classmates, and the college. Sophia's "Risks and Responsibilities" drawing (Figure 12.4) continues the softness of Figure 12.3 – Assistance, but now has a more defined identity: a mother bird gently eyeing four eggs to her right. She gazes with great tenderness and care, but the eggs appear vulnerable, just as taking responsibility and risks places Sophia in a vulnerable position.

12.2.4.1 Option One

By granting Kayla an extension to conduct the study over the summer, report actual data, and write the final chapters in her own words, Sophia fulfills her responsibility to Kayla by acknowledging Kayla's possible misunderstanding of the assignment and respects her honesty when Kayla admits to fabrication and plagiarism. As encouraged by literature indicating the importance of challenging academic misconduct (e.g., Hard et al., 2006; Keith-Spiegel et al., 2010), Sophia does not ignore Kayla's infractions, rather she makes an ethical decision to uphold the college's policies on flexibility in rectifying academic dishonesty.

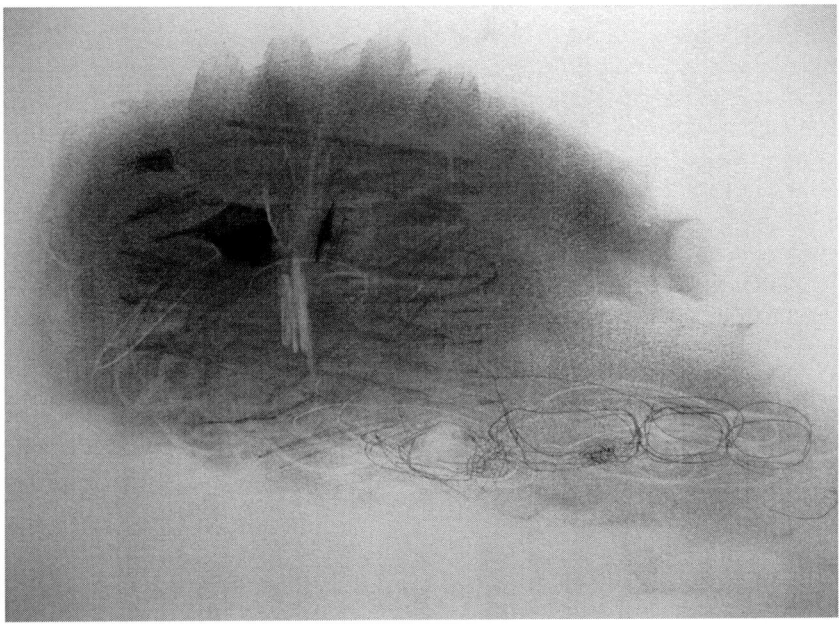

Figure 12.4 Responsibility & risks – A soft creature shelters fragile and un-
hatched eggs.

Sophia might fulfill her responsibility to Gabrielle by recognizing that
if Option One is chosen, Gabrielle may continue to receive services from
Kayla beyond the agreed-upon timeframe for the internship. However, by
not applying the full penalty for Kayla's infractions, Sophia might run
the risk of putting undue pressure on Gabrielle to provide oversight into
the summer. Further, Sophia does not fulfill her responsibility to the
college and the profession because she would be ignoring the ethical
standards expected of art therapists and art therapy educators.

12.2.4.2 Option Two

In Option Two, Sophia fulfills her ethical responsibility and reduces her
liability to concerned parties. However, it is possible Kayla will retaliate
by bringing her case to the Academic Grievance Committee. Nonetheless,
by reporting the academic dishonesty and assigning a failing grade,
Sophia fulfills her responsibility for fairness to students, and to the college
by implementing the academic integrity guidelines. Sophia also fulfills her
responsibility Gabrielle because the internship contract is honored and
there is no pressure to continue supervising Kayla beyond the internship's
final day.

12.2.5 T-Take Action

After considering all aspects of the case, Sophia selects Option Two as the most ethical action to take. By assigning a failing grade, Sophia would be upholding ATCB (2021) codes 1.3.2, 1.4, 2.7 as well as American Art Therapy Association (2013) principles 8.1 and 10.8. Further, Sophia would comply with the institution's academic integrity policy, not pressure Gabrielle to provide supervision beyond the bounds of the original internship, and would prevent a situation of undue treatment. This option is also supported by literature and consultants. Finally, Sophia would be fulfilling her responsibility to Gabrielle, the college, and the profession of art therapy. Option 2 is illustrated in Figure 12.5 which depicts a series of firm, solid, and bounded shapes. It consists of a large outside square containing a small square which contains a large circle and a small, barely visible, bright, white circle. The solidity of the inner square depicts Sophia's resolve and determination to Take Action. It protects the larger and small inner circles and substantially decreases feelings of vulnerability. The sequence of geometric shapes is balanced, complementary, and visually integrated.

12.2.5.1 Post-Case Follow-Up

In implementing Option 2, Sophia informs Kayla that, in compliance with the college's policy and procedures on academic integrity, she is required to report the situation and apply a failing grade to Kayla's thesis course. Sophia writes a report about the incident which is submitted and accepted by the college's dean, and placed in Kayla's academic file. Subsequently, Kayla registers for the course in order to graduate the following year.

12.3 Summary of the Main Concerns

There are several main concerns in ensuring the ethical conduct of research. First, to what degree do practitioners balance academic integrity policies and procedures, ethical principles of the American Art Therapy Association (2013), and ethical codes of the Art Therapy Credential Board (2021). While these are often in alignment, sometimes they conflict requiring art therapists to further process a dilemma. A second main concern involves weighing the seriousness of a research ethics violation and its potential implications on the field. Finally, the ethical conduct of research requires researchers to be competent. Consequently, it is important to provide opportunities for art therapists interested in research to gain a mastery of research methods, practices, and ethics.

12.4 Tips for Avoiding Pitfalls

To avoid research ethics violations, art therapists need to stay up to date with research ethics standards, principles, and codes in art therapy as well

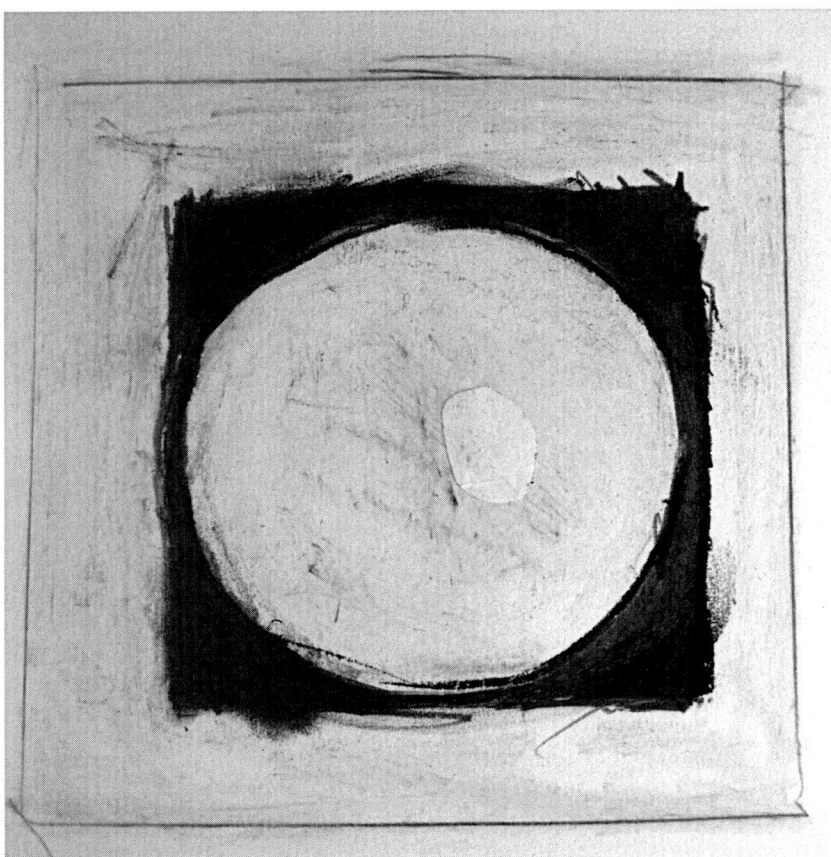

Figure 12.5 Take action – Calm, focus, and direction.

as related fields (e.g., psychology; counseling). Professional associations periodically revise their research ethics statements and this may affect art therapists conducting research. Further, art therapists should gain familiarity with state and federal regulations governing research. In addition, prior to writing a research proposal, researchers should consult with their Institutional Review Board (IRB) regarding their ethical codes and required documentation for research with human participants. For example, medical institutions frequently have extremely rigorous ethical standards and protocols, and their review process often takes months. As such, it's important to check with the IRB about time frames and requirements for submitting a research proposal, and submit the IRB's required proposal application form well in advance of the starting date of a study. It may also be beneficial to take an ethics training course and there are a variety of options available.

Another relevant issue involves gathering informed consent. This consent must be given by an adult, aged 18 or older. The adult may be a potential participant in the study, the parent or guardian of a participant (usually a minor), or an adult-in-need-of-assistance due to a medical or other condition. Best practices involve collecting assent from a child or adolescent to participate in the study. In seeking consent and/or assent, researchers must be completely transparent and inform the potential participant about everything they will be expected to do, without using deceptive practices. These forms should be written in language participants, parents, or guardians understand, and they should be offered the opportunity to ask questions. Art therapy researchers should also use an Artwork Release Form to obtain permission to photograph or in some way retain a record of the artwork.

Confidentiality is also a key component in the ethical practice of research. Efforts should be made to ensure participant identity and records are only accessible to those who need access. Whenever possible, anonymity in participant data should be preserved. For example, researchers may separate identifying information from participant responses, use a pseudonym for case studies, or not collect identifying information beyond what is needed for IRB. For artwork, researchers should delete or mask participants' names, signatures, or other identifying material on the artwork and in other places. Similarly, researchers should not photograph, videotape, or audiotape participants without their explicit, signed permission. Researchers should also keep in mind that participants can withdraw this permission at any time without repercussions and this information should be included on the consent or assent form.

Finally, researchers need to ensure they are competent. For those not trained in research they should consider taking a course or courses, including a statistics course, working on a research project(s) with a colleague or mentor, and consulting with a researcher who regularly conducts studies. It may also be beneficial to read research studies on topics that interest you in other professional journals in addition to art therapy journals to become familiar with the various research methodologies, how they are applied, and the structure, sequence, and rigor of research studies. Asking an experienced researcher to read a research proposal prior to submitting it to the IRB can help to avoid ethical concerns arising in the IRB review phase. As always, art therapists are encouraged to make artwork to better navigate and process personal and professional challenges.

12.5 Suggested Further Readings

Betts, D. J. & Deaver, S. P. (2019). *Art therapy research: A practical guide*. Routledge.

This volume is a comprehensive and thorough examination of quantitative, qualitative, arts-based, and mixed methods research. It provides thorough coverage of the literature available for each methodology. In addition, the book includes exercises that will engage readers in direct application of several research methods including research ethics.

Corts, D. P., & Tatum, H. E. (2019). *Ethics in psychological research: A practical guide for the student scientist.* Sage.

This volume is essential reading for all researchers and covers all aspects of ethical research. Of particular relevance are the chapters on research misconduct and ethical writing practices which cover falsification, fabrication, and plagiarism. Each chapter is similarly structured. Beginning with a research dilemma and discussion of the broader topic, including additional examples from the authors' experiences, the chapters conclude with a summary, discussion questions, and additional resources.

Farrant, C., Pavlicevic, M., & Tsiris, G. (2014). *A guide to research ethics for arts therapists and arts & healthcare practitioners.* Jessica Kingsley Publishers.

This book covers research ethics for allied health professions. The book beings by placing research ethics in context, before moving on to essential topics common to all research: Responsibility to research participants, including a discussion of confidentiality, anonymity, and privacy, informed consent or assent, usage of data, including demographic data, and preparing a proposal for the Institutional Review Board (IRB), or Research Ethics Committee (REC). The volume is replete with practical and real-life applications, resources, and suggested readings.

Kapitan, L. (2018). *An introduction to art therapy research* (2nd ed.). Routledge.

Kapitan (2018) discusses finding a research question, the role of art, ethics, writing a research report, and writing for publication. She discusses the boundaries of conducting studies, uses of art as data, as well as identifying areas where ethical misconduct might occur: Multiple Roles, Confidentiality, Informed Consent, and Deception and Disclosure. She brings in ethical thinking from multiple sources, placing ethical art therapy research practice akin to those of allied fields. A sample of a consent form is provided as a model of transparency and an example of the depth of a study's description in order to avoid deceptive practice.

Pope, K. S., & Vasquez, M. J. T. (2011). *Ethics in psychotherapy and counseling: A practical guide* (4th ed.). John Wiley & Sons. https://doi.org/10.1002/9781118001875

Pope and Vasquez's book is a classic in the field. Although the authors cover many topics related to psychotherapy and counseling, they address research ethics in several sections, and their teachings are generalizable to the field of art therapy and other helping professions. Informed consent and assent are required before participants engage in taking assessments. Reporting data accurately and maintaining a record of raw data is essential in research studies. When testing occurs in research, the assessment protocol must be followed exactly as written, and each participant must be assessed in exactly the same way. Cultural competence is required both in therapy and research. These are just a few concerns in which research ethics and ethical behavior in counseling overlap. Finally, multiple relationships occur when the therapist is also the researcher. Attention to the boundaries and demands of each relationship is central to ethics in research as well as treatment. Their stance is that research ethics permeate every aspect of research studies.

References

American Art Therapy Association. (2013). *Ethical principles for art therapists*. https://arttherapy.org/wp-content/uploads/2017/06/Ethical-Principles-for-Art-Therapists.pdf

Art Therapy Credentials Board. (2021). *Code of ethics, conduct, and disciplinary procedures*. https://www.atcb.org/wp-content/uploads/2020/07/ATCB-Code-of-Ethics-Conduct-DisciplinaryProcedures.pdf

Betts, D. J., & Deaver, S. P. (2019). *Art therapy research: A practical guide*. Routledge. 10.4324/9781315647081

Columbia University. (n.d.). *RCR research misconduct*. https://ccnmtl.columbia.edu/projects/rcr/rcr_misconduct/foundation/index.html

Corts, D. P., & Tatum, H. E. (2019). *Ethics in psychological research: A practical guide for the student scientist*. Sage. 10.4135/9781544345352

Daniel-McKeigue, C. J. (2007). Cracking the code: What are the ethical implications of designing a research study that relates to therapeutic interventions with children in play therapy? *The Arts in Psychotherapy, 34*(3), 238–248. 10.1016/j.aip.2007.02.001

Farrant, C., Pavlicevic, M., & Tsiris, G. (2014). *A guide to research ethics for arts therapists and arts and healthcare practitioners*. Jessica Kingsley Publishers.

Hard, S. F., Conway, J. M., & Moran, A. C. (2006). Faculty and college student beliefs about the frequency of student academic misconduct. *The Journal of Higher Education, 77*(6), 1058–1080. 10.1353/jhe.2006.0048

Jordan, A. E. (2010). College student cheating: The role of motivation, perceived norms, attitudes, and knowledge of institutional policy. *Ethics & Behavior, 11*(3), 233–247. 10.1207/s15327019eb1103_3

Kapitan, L. (2018). *An introduction to art therapy research* (2nd ed.). Routledge. 10.4324/9781315691749

Keith-Spiegel, P., Tabachnick, B. G., Whitley Jr., B. E., & Washburn, J. (2010). Why professors ignore cheating: Opinions of a national sample of psychology instructors. *Ethics & Behavior, 8*(3), 215–227. 10.1207/s15327019eb0803_3

LaBeff, E. E., Clark, R. E., Haines, V. J., & Diekhoff, G. M. (1990). Situational ethics and college student cheating. *Sociological Inquiry, 60*(7), 190–198. 10.1111/j.1475-682X.1990.tb00138.x

Lau, K. K., & Huag, J. C. (2011). The impact of sex, college, major, and student classification on students' perception of ethics. *Mustang Journal of Business &*

Ethics, *2*, 86–99. http://mustangjournals.com/MJBE/v2_MJBE_2011_ forwebsite.pdf#page=86

Meng, C. L., Othman, J., D'Silva, J. L., & Omar, Z. (2014). Ethical decision making in academic dishonesty with application of modified theory of planned behavior: A review. *International Education Studies*, *7*(3), 126–139.

National Institutes of Health. (2021, March). *Ethics in clinical research.* https:// clinicalcenter.nih.gov/recruit/ethics.html

Stearns, S. A. (2010). The student-instructor relationship's effect on academic integrity. *Ethics & Behavior*, *11*(3), 275–285. 10.1207/S15327019EB1103_6

13 Ethical Decision-Making as a Valuable Clinical Tool

Jessica M. Hauck and Thomson J. Ling

The *Ethical Principles for Art Therapists* starts with the idea that "art therapists endeavor to advance the welfare of their clients" (American Art Therapy Association, 2013, p. 2). In general terms, this can be translated into a call for art therapists to help others. However, this desire to help others can often create a blind spot when it comes to ethical decision-making. In ensuring ethical practice, it is important to note that practitioners are evaluated by their actions and not their intentions. Indeed, a well-intentioned action can sometimes be a slippery slope that creates ethical quandaries.

The DO ART model provides practitioners with a pathway to start to think through the ethical challenges in art therapy (Hauck & Ling, 2016, 2020). This process can be challenging and intimidating for clinicians of all experience levels. Having an approachable model to work through ethical dilemmas is one way clinicians can set themselves up for success in this area. Art therapists possess unique critical thinking skills, which creates an opportunity to blend different approaches of thinking (visual and verbal) to work through these dilemmas in a more effective way.

As art therapists are aware, art is a powerful tool for processing and externalizing. The inherent containment in an art-making process has the benefit of making a decision-making process manageable and less overwhelming. Moreover, using art in the ethical decision-making process allows art therapists to utilize their strengths by incorporating a set of prescribed visualizations to navigate a process that is traditionally emotionally closed off and staunchly logical. The DO ART model was designed to be approachable for art therapists in training, practicing art therapists, and other practitioners that may be visual and kinesthetic learners.

13.1 Strengths and Limitations of the DO ART Model

The DO ART model takes various theoretical perspectives into consideration in the decision-making process and is applicable to a broad variety of art therapy situations. This model encourages best practices by

DOI: 10.4324/9781003175124-13

incorporating recent relevant literature. At one point, practitioners had argued against linear models in favor of ones that consider clients in the specific context of their situation (Meara et al., 1996; Rave & Larsen, 1995); the DO ART model balances these two perspectives by providing a linear model that also considers the context in which practitioners are making the decision.

Despite the length of the model, many of the steps can be done quickly with clear progression, because of the linear and logical organization. As art therapists use the model and grow more familiar with it, the steps can also be quickly applied to situations where split-second decisions must be made. While many existing ethical decision-making models assume that practitioners understand how to identify an ethical dilemma without providing a clear explanation, the DO ART model provides a clear and comprehensive process for understanding the ethical dilemma, so that practitioners with all levels of experience can apply the model confidently.

13.2 Empirical Evidence for the Effectiveness of the DO ART Model

Since the field of art therapy is constantly growing and evolving, it is important to provide empirical evidence supporting the tools that art therapists use, including ethical decision-making models. Despite the availability of many ethical decision-making models (e.g., Corey et al., 2015; Forester-Miller & Davis, 1996; Frame & Williams, 2005; Hill & Mamalakis, 2001; Sileo & Kopala, 1993), there has been a lack of literature investigating the effectiveness of models. With the emergence of the DO ART model, the field of art therapy became the leader in examining the effectiveness of ethical decision-making models.

In a recently published study (Ling et al., 2019), the DO ART model was compared with an established model of ethical decision-making (i.e., Sileo & Kopala, 1993). This study examined a collection of student papers that applied an ethical decision-making model to a case vignette (Hauck & Ling, 2016; Sileo & Kopala, 1993).

Four outcome measures were developed reflecting different aspects of ethical decision-making to assess the effectiveness of the models: Obligations were the degree to which a deontological framework was included, specifically, if the established rules that govern behavior are adhered to such that liability is limited. Moral Ideals referred to the consideration of common principle ethics and spoke to a moral relativism framework. Specifically, this includes autonomy, beneficence, non-maleficence, justice, veracity, and fidelity. Consequences were the degree to which a utilitarian perspective was used to examine the results of considered courses of action. Finally, Bias referred to whether decisions were made prematurely without considering the various aspects of ethical decision-making. Each measure was rated on a four-point scale where one represented an absence of the criteria and four indicated that the criteria were included, considered, and weighed in the decision-making process.

The results of this study indicate that art therapists are as effective as practitioners in counseling-related fields in the use of ethical decision-making models and in considering all four aspects of ethical decision-making. In addition, it was found that the DO ART model is as effective as existing ethical decision-making models on these four dimensions of ethical decision-making. While the study examined graduate students rather than professional art therapists, it is likely that practicing art therapists may be equally or more effective in using ethical decision-making models. Nonetheless, to our knowledge, this is the first study to examine the effectiveness of any ethical decision-making models and provides evidence of the utility of the DO ART model. We believe that the evidence behind the DO ART model encourages evidenced-based practice, and furthers the profession by reinforcing the use of art as both a treatment modality and a resource for ethical professional development.

13.3 Common Challenges using the DO ART Model

While the DO ART Model provides practitioners with a framework for organizing the ethical decision-making process in creative art therapies, there are some challenges that therapists commonly face when becoming familiar with the model. In applying the Dilemma step, practitioners sometimes forget to consider the ethical codes and principles in their totality. That is, occasionally art therapists will focus on one section of the code of ethics, laws, or ethical principles and not consider how other sections may be relevant to the situation being analyzed. Further, in identifying the dilemma, while good ethical decision-making is about looking forward, practitioners may be tempted to use the DO ART model to identify missteps that have already occurred. While being able to identify past missteps is incredibly important for the prevention of future ethical challenges, focusing on decisions that have already been made and outcomes that have already occurred may not allow practitioners to adequately analyze the courses of action going forward in order to reach a resolution to the identified ethical dilemma.

In the Outcomes step, we caution art therapists against looking at outcomes too narrowly, by only focusing on the art therapists and the client. While the clinician and the client are typically the most affected by an ethical dilemma, it is important to acknowledge that art therapy practice does not occur separately from outside events and influences (i.e., it does not occur in a vacuum). Actions taken and decisions made by an art therapist may have far-reaching consequences that affect other parties. Therefore, in applying the DO ART model, clinicians should be sure to consider how actions taken to resolve a dilemma may affect other parties. Similarly, art therapists may not always parse the implications of a course of action by option and by party but rather focus on only one dimension (i.e., option or party). It is important that outcomes be parsed by option considered and by the party affected. Put another way, art therapists should calculate the probability that an action taken may have desirable outcomes for some parties but not others.

Assistance consists of two parts: assistance from people and assistance from the literature. A common challenge in receiving Assistance from people is the temptation for an art therapist to offload a decision to a consultant. Some practitioners may even apply for Assistance from people step by polling a variety of consultants about what to do. Put another way, it can be tempting to simply ask others to make the decision for us (i.e., pass the buck). We caution art therapists from using Assistance in this way because it does not allow an art therapist to combine input from consultants to the decision-making process. In addition, allowing consultants to make a decision may place an art therapist at risk given that the art therapist and not the consultant hold liability for the ethical decision being made. In receiving assistance from the literature, a common challenge is ensuring the appropriateness of the literature. We remind art therapists that the purpose of reviewing the literature is to ensure that ethical decisions are made in the context of current practice and that decisions are in alignment with industry standards. As a result, it is important for art therapists to ensure that the literature they are considering is current (i.e., recent) and not an outlier (i.e., a fringe opinion). In other words, we suggest that art therapists consider multiple sources of recent, relevant information.

The Risk step is an area where art therapists often have difficulty differentiating from other steps when applying the model. While this section considers similar relevant parties to the Outcomes step, the Risk step is a separate and distinct step. The outcomes step of the DO ART model uses a utilitarian approach to consider what is the greatest good for the most number of people, whereas the Risk step focuses on the art therapist and their exposure to risk from these various parties. Put another way, the Risk step focuses on the potential for an ethics complaint or lawsuit to be brought against an art therapist. Since ethics complaints and lawsuits can come from multiple parties, clinicians consider the same constituents they did in the outcome step but are less concerned with benefit to these parties in the Risk step.

A final challenge art therapists encounter is not ending the DO ART model by actually taking action that follows from the previous steps. Art therapists may reach the end of the model and find the most ethical/least unethical course of action does not agree with their gut instinct. We believe that the ethical decision-making model should be used to reach a decision about a pathway forward rather than be used to justify a prematurely selected course of action. We remind art therapists that good ethical decision-making involves making a logical decision and taking the best course of action even if it may not align with gut instincts, which are emotional by nature. This is not to say that practitioners should ignore emotions, rather than one's gut instinct should never supersede a well-applied decision-making process.

13.4 The Place of the DO ART Model in Practice

While the DO ART Model provides practitioners with a valuable tool for ethical decision-making, it is important to note that this model rests within a larger context of ethical practice. In addition to being able to apply a decision-making model, the ethical practice includes Intentionality, Moral principles, Knowledge of laws and professional standards, Self-Awareness, and personal convictions (Remley & Herlihy, 2020). Intentionality includes approaching practice with the goal of acting within professional ethics. Moral principles include an awareness of one's own moral compass as well as the moral compass of the profession. Knowledge of laws and professional standards involves being familiar with the various laws, regulations, and practicing standards of one's jurisdiction. Self-awareness involves understanding how one's personal beliefs and values may affect their approach to an ethical dilemma. Finally, personal convictions involve acting with a high level of integrity regardless of potential negative personal impacts. As art therapists gain familiarity and use the DO ART model, we remind practitioners that these other aspects of ethical practice continue to play a role in informing decision-making.

13.5 Concluding Thoughts

As we conclude this book, we are reminded of our mothers who, in childhood, responded to our poor decisions by saying, "I am not interested in your intentions, I am interested in your behaviors." As we have become practitioners, we have often thought about how we can act in a way that aligns our behaviors and our intentions in a way that provides the best outcomes for all parties. The DO ART model provides guidance for acting ethically in art therapy; however, it is important to note that the practice of art therapy affects individuals and ethical decisions need to keep in mind. We believe that by gaining familiarity with ethical decision-making, art therapists can ensure that, when faced with ambiguous dilemmas, they are fulfilling both their ethical responsibilities while simultaneously ensuring the actions they take are helpful to their clients.

References

American Art Therapy Association. (2013). *Ethical principles for art therapists.* https://arttherapy.org/wp-content/uploads/2017/06/Ethical-Principles-for-Art-Therapists.pdf

Corey, G., Corey, M. S., & Callanan, P. (2015). *Issues and ethics in the helping professions* (9th ed.). Brooks/Cole.

Forester-Miller, H., & Davis, T. (1996). *A practitioner's guide to ethical decision making*. American Counseling Association. http://www.counseling.org/docs/ethics/practitioners_guide.pdf?sfvrsn=2

Frame, M. W., & Williams, C. B. (2005). A model of ethical decision making from a multicultural perspective. *Counseling and Values, 49*(3), 165–179. 10.1002/j.21 61-007X.2005.tb01020.x

Hauck, J., & Ling, T. (2016). The DO ART model: An ethical decision-making model applicable to art therapy. *Art Therapy: Journal of the American Art Therapy Association, 33*(4), 203–208. 10.1080/07421656.2016.1231544

Hauck, J.M., & Ling, T.J. (2020). Applying art therapy directives to ethical decision-making. *Art Therapy: Journal of the American Art Therapy Association, 37*(1), 34–41. 10.1080/07421656.2019.1667669

Hill, M.R., & Mamalakis, P.M. (2001). Family therapists and religious communities: Negotiating dual relationships. *Family Relations, 50*(3), 199–208. 10.1111/j.1741-3729.2001.00199.x

Ling, T. J., Hauck, J. M., Doyle, C. J., Percario, K. N., & Henawi, T. (2019). Evaluating the use of ethical decision-making models for art therapy. *Art Therapy: Journal of the American Art Therapy Association, 36*(2), 93–97 10.1080/07421656.2019.1609330

Meara, N. M., Schmidt, L. D., & Day, J. D. (1996). Principles and virtues: A foundation for ethical decisions, policies, and character. *The Counseling Psychologist, 24*, 4–77. 10.1177/0011000096241002

Rave, E. J., & Larsen, C. C. (1995). *Ethical decision-making in therapy: Feminist perspectives*. Guilford Press.

Remley, T. P., & Herlihy, B. (2020). *Ethical, legal, and professional issues in counseling* (6th ed.). Pearson.

Sileo, F.J., & Kopala, M. (1993). An A-B-C-D-E worksheet for promoting beneficence when considering ethical issues. *Counseling and Values, 37*(2), 89–95. 10.1002/j.2161-007X.1993.tb00800.x

Index